WHO GETS HEALTH CARE?

An Arena for Nursing Action

Editor

Barbara Kos-Munson, Ph.D., R.N., C.S., a founding editor of *Scholarly Inquiry for Nursing Practice,* is currently a Professor Emeritus at Adelphi University in Garden City, NY. For 18 years she served in both teaching and administration positions in the School of Nursing, assuming the roles of Director of the Doctoral Program, Associate Dean, and Acting Dean. Having graduated from the Postdoctorate Program in Psychoanalysis and Psychotherapy, she left in 1987 to concentrate on full-time private practice.

Dr. Kos-Munson was recipient of an American Research Grant in Aid, studying recovery post-coronary bypass surgery. She has been both officer and board member of the American Heart Association Nassau Region and Pederson-Krag Mental Health Center. She has been honored by the Long Island Professional Women's Association, receiving their award in Health Care and by Adelphi University as their distinguished alumna 1986.

Editors of *Scholarly Inquiry for Nursing Practice*

WHO GETS HEALTH CARE?

An Arena for Nursing Action

Barbara Kos-Munson
Editor

SPRINGER PUBLISHING COMPANY
New York

Copyright © 1993 by Springer Publishing Company, Inc.

All right reserved

No part of this publication may be reproduced, stored in a retrieval system, or transmitted in any form or by any means electronic, mechanical, photocopying, recording, or otherwise, without the prior permission of Springer Publishing Company, Inc.

Springer Publishing Company, Inc.
536 Broadway
New York, NY 10012

94 95 96 97 / 5 4 3

Library of Congress Cataloging-in-Publication Data

Who gets health care? : an arena for nursing action / Barbara Kos-Munson, editor.
    p.   cm.
    Includes bibliographical references
    ISBN 0-8261-8240-2
    1. Right to health care—United States. 2. Medical policy—United States.
    3. Nurses—United States—Political activity. I. Kos-Munson, Barbara.
    [DNLM: 1. Delivery of Health Care—United States. 2. Health Policy—
    United States. 3. Nursing—trends—United States. WY16 W6373]
RA395.A3W485 1993
362. 1'0973—dc 20
DNLM/DLC
for Library of Congress   92-48981
                                                   CIP

Printed in the United States of America

Contents

Contributors

Peter S. Arno, Ph.D., is an Associate Professor in the Department of Epidemiology and Social Medicine at the Montefiore Medical Center, Einstein College of Medicine, New York. He received his doctorate in economics from the New School for Social Research, and was a postdoctoral research fellow at the Institute for Health Policy Studies and the Institute for Health and Aging at the University of California, San Francisco. Arno is a renowned author, researcher, and speaker on major issues and problems including economics of health care, AIDS, substance abuse, and homelessness. He is a co-author of the new book, *Against the Odds: The Story of AIDS, Drug Development, Politics & Profits.*

Mila Aroskar, Ed.D., R.N., F.A.A.N., is Associate Professor in the Division of Health Services Administration at the School of Public Health, and Faculty Associate at the Center for Biomedical Ethics, University of Minnesota, Minneapolis. She received her doctorate in curriculum development from the State University of New York at Buffalo. She is a former Joseph P. Kennedy, Jr. Fellow in Medical Ethics, Harvard University. Aroskar is a noted author, lecturer and consultant on ethics in nursing and health care, recently co-authoring *Ethical Dilemmas and Nursing Practice, 3rd Ed.*

Virginia Trotter Betts, M.S.N., J.D., R.N., is a Research Associate Professor and Senior Research Associate at the Vanderbilt University Institute for Public Policy Studies. Her varied educational background, first in psychiatric-mental health nursing and then in law, led her to postdoctoral study in health policy at the Institute of Medicine, National Academy of Sciences in Washington. Betts is a noted consultant, lecturer and author of more than 50 articles and books on topics combining nursing and law. She has been extremely active in A.N.A. affairs, currently holding the position of President.

Karen A. Bonuck, M.P.A., M.S.W., is a Research Associate in the Department of Epidemiology and Social Medicine at Montefiore Medical Center, and Adjunct Field Instructor at the Columbia University School of Social Work in New York. She had previously served as Health Policy Analyst in the New Jersey Department of Human Services and the New York City Health and Hospitals Corporation. Her M.P.A. and M.S.W. were earned at Columbia University, and she has completed all course work for a Ph.D. in Social Work at Rutgers University. The title of her dissertation, in progress, is "Prevalence of, and Factors Associated with, Unmet Needs in Persons with AIDS and HIV Illness."

3

Carolyne K. Davis, Ph.D., R.N., currently serves as a national consultant to the firm of Ernst & Young. She holds a master's degree in nursing education and a doctorate in higher education administration. Having served as Dean of the School of Nursing at the University of Michigan, she soon assumed broader administrative duties as Associate Vice President for Academic Affairs. From 1981 through 1985, Davis served as Administrator of the Health Care Financing Administration (HCFA) of the Department of Health and Human Services, overseeing health care services for 54 million disadvantaged, disabled, and elderly Americans. She has published widely on issues related to the health care system.

Lucille A. Joel, Ed.D., R.N., F.A.A.N., as immediate past President of the American Nurses Association, was for four years the official representative of two million registered nurses and the organization's spokesperson on public policy. She is recognized nationally as a health care leader, having appeared on network television and been interviewed by major newspapers and magazines. Joel continues as Professor and Chair in the Department of Adults and the Aged at Rutgers University's College of Nursing, and is gubernatorial appointee to the Health Care Administration Board of New Jersey.

Joel S. Levine, M.D., is currently Associate Dean for Hospital Affairs at the School of Medicine, University of Colorado, and President of the medical staff of University Hospital. His educational background includes an M.D. from SUNY Downstate Medical Center, New York, with a specialty in internal medicine, and studies at the Tufts-New England Medical Center, in gastroenterology, and at the University of Colorado Health Sciences Center. As health legislative aide to Senator Max Baucus of Montana, Levine helped to design rural health legislation that passed in the Budget Reconciliation Act of 1989. He continued as aide to Senator Baucus, who served on the Pepper Commission. Levine's expertise in matters of health care delivery, particularly in rural areas, is well recognized.

Patricia Moccia, Ph.D., R.N., F.A.A.N., is Executive Vice President of the National League for Nursing and Vice President of Education and Accreditation, overseeing N.L.N.'s multilevel educational, accreditation, and consultation services. She is also an Adjunct Professor at the Union for Experimenting Colleges and Universities. Her educational credentials include undergraduate, master's, and doctoral degrees in nursing from New York University. Moccia has held a number of academic positions including Chair of the Department of Nursing Education at Teachers College, Columbia University and Adjunct Associate Professor at the Baruch College School of Business and Public Administration in New York. In the public policy arena, she serves on the Advisory Committee of Medical Services for the Homeless with the Community for Creative Non-Violence in Washington, D.C., and she has authored many articles related to health care delivery.

James L. Muyskens, Ph.D., is Dean of the College of Liberal Arts and Sciences, University of Kansas. He received his Ph.D. in philosophy from the University of Michigan and his M. Div. from Princeton Theological Seminary. Following graduation, Muyskens was appointed to a faculty position, culminating in a promotion to Acting Provost at Hunter College, New York. Muysken's interest and expertise in the area of nursing and health care ethics is made abundantly clear by his authorship of dozens of articles on the collective responsibility of nurses, nurses' right to strike, and the just allocation of scarce medical resources. His book, *Moral Problems in Nursing: A Philosophical Investigation*, was published in 1990.

Patricia Stevens, R.N., Ph.D., is a postdoctoral fellow at the University of California at San Francisco (UCSF). Her fellowship is funded by a National Research Service Award from the National Center for Nursing Research. Her research is about lesbians living with Human Immunodeficiency Virus (HIV), specifically their acess to health care services, interactions with health care providers, and self-care practices. Stevens's work has so far resulted in more than 20 articles and book chapters.

Introduction

In preparing this book on health care access, which originated as a special issue of *Scholarly Inquiry for Nursing Practice*, my thoughts went back to a time 20 years ago when I taught my first graduate course—a course focused on health care policy and delivery. It was, and continues to be, a topic holding enormous interest for me. I struggled to put together all of the topical materials available at the time from medical, sociological, cultural, psychological, philosophic, and media sources. At that time, there was apparently little interest in research or theory building related to health care delivery in any of the disciplines. With very few exceptions, nursing literature on the topic was nonexistent.

Since then, public interest literature in health care delivery in every professional field, and rhetoric, if not accompanying action, has increased one-hundred-fold. The media message is most often a negative one, while the professional literature presents, at best, a mixed picture. Government officials and government hopefuls are making health care a hot election topic and a rallying cry of the '90s. Meanwhile, nursing has just begun to take the more assertive role in forming health care policy that it has more typically taken in delivering health care to individuals.

Stevens's premise in her encompassing lead chapter focuses on the fallibilities of our current methods of health care delivery, which leave perhaps 30% of our citizens uninsured or underinsured. As with business ventures, the system is driven by political and economic expediency and not by patient need. Often overlooked are the many who don't "qualify" as patients due to lack of insurance coverage, inadequate finances, age, both very young and very old, devastating chronic illness, "unacceptable" group membership, poor education or inability to communicate, and those needing "experimental" treatments. How can we as nurses continue to remain uninformed, disinterested, and silent?

Stevens follows up on the picture she has painted with the meaning of the term "equitable access," and a beginning conceptual framework within which nurses can work. She calls on each of us to fully embrace the notion of care for all through collective action, clinical practice, and research studies.

We chose outstanding representatives of varied disciplines and varied perspectives, both within and beyond nursing to respond to Stevens's chapter. What we hope to accomplish is to provide a forum for the knowledge, the beliefs, the thoughts, and the concerns of our authors, thereby promoting your thoughts and questions, your ideas, and your motivation to act.

Mila Aroskar responds to Stevens's paper, focusing directly on moral and ethical imperatives for nurses. She takes exception to Stevens's view that a mandate to ethical action is not in place, and goes on to examine the many societal and professional values that have focused our attention on the individual and not on "the good for all." Most important, Aroskar helps us to concentrate on the concept of justice in health care delivery, distinguishing among patient need, merit, and ability to pay, and on our personal responsibility to act on patients' behalf.

The focus of the response of Virginia Trotter Betts is the delineation of nursing's proposed policy for health care reform set out in *Nursing's Agenda for Health Care Reform.* She emphasizes the unique aspects of this package which go beyond ability to pay, and include geographical availability of providers as well as quality of care given to a complex mix of needy persons. Betts illustrates her response with examples of excellence and availability in care giving by nurses.

Karen Bonuck and Peter Arno, writing from a social policy perspective, acknowledge the contribution of nurses to health care delivery, at the same time citing nursing's failure to observe, document, and initiate changes where obstructions to access occur. They add to Stevens's argument for educational reform within the profession as part and parcel of the very early initiation and socialization of undergraduate students. The authors also argue for introducing young students to the political, economic, environmental, and social realities within which they will function as health care providers. A specific recommendation includes using the comprehensive Health Behavior Model as the lens through which to identify, analyze, and understand the factors limiting access to care. They urge that attention be paid to addressing the conflict between serving two masters—the patient, and the institution or system.

Carolyne Davis, in speaking from corporate or business as well as nursing perspectives, urges a look at the hard facts: we live in a country of people espousing health care ideals but unwilling to open their purses. Nurses, she contends, can do much to promote cost effectiveness in care, thereby allowing government, employers, and third-party payers to expand coverage. She points out that as desirable as alternative systems of care in other countries appear to be, costs and waiting time for care in these countries have risen rapidly. Finally, Davis calls for our responsible action in promoting high-quality, equitable health care for our citizens.

Lucille Joel highlights the irreconcilable dilemma in which we find ourselves as a profession, espousing promotion of health and prevention of illness while equal access to care is far from being a reality. At the same time, she cites an estimate of the projected health care bill for the year 2000 as $2.7 trillion. Indicative of careful deliberation and analyses, *Nursing's Agenda for Health Care Reform* was put forward as a plan that, according to Joel, is "realistic, practical, and based on first-hand understanding of what needs to be done." (A summary of *Nursing's Agenda for Health Care Reform* is included as an appendix in this issue.) She elaborates on provisions of the Agenda, including convenient access to managed care in schools and in the workplace, delivered by qualified professionals at an affordable price, paid for by reallocated dollars and not additional monies.

Reflecting a broad, political-economic focus, Joel Levine talks about the "fuzzy" messages that our legislators and executives receive from constituents, expressing dissatisfactions of all sorts regarding health care delivery, but with little unanimity on what should be done for whom, by whom, how, and at what cost. He reminds us of the powerful, opposing forces of advocacy groups and lobbyists who are better trained, better organized and better financed, thereby more effective in getting their messages across. Unfortunately, we compete for funds with other essential areas such as housing, education, and job training. Levine concludes his remarks with a look at delivery systems throughout the world and some lessons to be learned about cost containment, universal access, equality of coverage, and shared responsibility in a successful enterprise. He praises nurses' clinical work and public participation in helping to effect desired change.

Patricia Moccia focuses her response on the interrelationship or mediation of health care education and health care delivery, calling on both those areas to address the social construction and social function aspects of care delivery. She states further that reformation of system structures alone does not automatically address underlying societal beliefs and values. She asks us to consider the basic informing question, "qui bono?," or "to whose good?" It is Moccia's contention that what is called for in nursing education is the same depth of examination of social construction and social function of nursing practice as that undertaken both by Stevens and by nursing leaders who drew up *Nursing's Agenda for Health Care Reform.*

James Muyskens asks us to view health care in the United States through the eyes of an intergalactic traveler, puzzled by the dichotomy of amazing medical technology on the one hand and the many people untouched and ignored by the health care system on the other. As you begin to puzzle through the paradox he relates, you discover that our highly held values of individualism and egalitarianism have mitigated against equal access to health care. He contends that "rationing" of services occurs because of limitations of finances as well as of staff and space. In departure from Stevens's call for a revised system of care providing equitable access, Muyskens's more modest goal is the provision of a "decent minimum" of care for all. He raises the notion of a utopian dream versus realistic limits and fairness to all. Both he and Stevens concur that nurses collectively can and must play a part in reformulating priorities and goals.

Several thoughts occurred to me while summarizing the valuable contributions of each of our authors. Varying perspectives enrich and inform us and prompt us to question and to weigh alternatives. My thoughts led me to consider the "haves and have nots," those designated as "patients" and those others deemed "nonpatients," or "unpatients" or "a-patients." It's interesting to note that, according to *Webster's New World Dictionary,* the noun "patient" is derived from the same Latin and Old French roots, meaning "to suffer." The quality of being patient requires "bearing or enduring pain, trouble, without complaining or losing control or making a disturbance," while to be a patient means to be "a person receiving care or treatment, especially under the care of a doctor." Most would agree that to be a patient requires one to be patient. What, then, of a nonpatient? Is the requirement impatience? Super-patience? Or does being a nonpatient merely manifest itself in chronic illness, continuation of a welfare legacy, hopelessness and despair? It's well past time to understand the meaning of being excluded from minimal basic care and to act on this injustice.

All of our authors have urged change. Several concur with Stevens on the nature of that change, which would include a radical revision of the existing system. Others have focused on specific aspects for change. Propositions differ in both kind and degree. Lofty ideals, while not usually possible to attain, do serve to guide us. Despite the slowness of change and our collective impatience and sometimes discouragement, we cannot afford to forsake our dream of access for all. For as Virginia Woolf reminded us over 60 years ago, "He who robs us of our dreams, robs us of our life" (Orlando, 203).

Barbara A. Kos-Munson, Ph.D., R.N., C.S.

1

Who Gets Care?
Access to Health Care as an Arena
for Nursing Action

Patricia E. Stevens, R.N., Ph.D.

School of Nursing
University of California, San Francisco

Access to health care in the United States is undeniably inequitable. What should nurses do in the face of increasing gaps in availability of services? The author addresses this question by framing access to health care in its broadest sociopolitical context, positing that access to care is an essential dimension of nursing theory, research, and practice. By offering a conceptual definition of equitable access, providing rationale for the significance of this concept, and critically exploring conditions that limit access to affordable, high quality, nondiscriminatory health care in the U.S., the author lays theoretical groundwork for more effective investigatory and practical action to assure equitable access.

The American Nurses Association's (1980) *Nursing: A Social Policy Statement* states that nursing is accountable for the accessibility of health care. Even though nurses have had this mandate for more than a decade, there is little evidence that actions to assure accessibility have entered our practice, research, and theory in a significant way. To become well informed about access to health care services, one must read widely outside disciplinary boundaries. The inequity of health care access in the United States has been the focus of several recent contributions to the nursing literature (Cohen, 1990; Davis, 1988; Dimond, 1989; Funkhouser & Moser, 1990; Hall & Stevens, 1991; Harrington, 1988, 1990; Hodnicki, 1990; MacPherson, 1987, 1989; Martin & Henry, 1989; Mitchell, Krueger, & Moody, 1990; Moccia, 1988; Moccia & Mason, 1986; Rooks, 1990; Ross, 1989; Smith, 1990). Nursing, however, has come late to the table of discontent regarding current systems of health care distribution.

Why has nursing not incorporated access to care as a central phenomenon of investigative and practical significance? By ignoring access as a focal element of nursing theory, research, and practice, we effectively give up our power to impact the structures and policies that determine availability of health care. Without universal access to adequate care, nursing may eventually become a luxury

11

affordable by only a dominant, affluent class of health care consumers. If nursing shies away from an aggressively critical exploration of health care access in the United States, it will be relegated to politically ineffectual, subservient roles in the health care arena, capable of providing care, but voiceless in terms of who gets that care.

Nursing practice is grounded in values of caring (Benner & Wrubel, 1988; Leininger, 1988; Paterson & Zderad, 1976; Watson, 1985) and advocacy for vulnerable populations (American Nurses Association Cabinet on Nursing Research, 1985). Nurses have intimate clinical knowledge of the full spectrum of health services delivery: the minute details of hands-on care, the suffering of clients and their significant others, the institutional constraints under which care is provided, and the practices of other health care providers. Nurses are in a strategic position to document and criticize the interactional, structural, and ideological circumstances that impede clients' access to and positive experience of health care.

Too often, in our attempts to suggest solutions to everyday health problems, nurses address only individual health behaviors, while overlooking glaring social, economic, and political conditions that are detrimental to the population's health (Butterfield, 1990; MacPherson, 1987). The notion of individual motivation and responsibility is a cherished and pervasive value in North American society, but one which often leads to victim-blaming ideologies in the human sciences (Funkhouser & Moser, 1990; Kidder & Fine, 1986; Milio, 1988; Ryan, 1971; Seidman & Rappaport, 1986; Williams, 1989). Without reframing nursing theory and research about clients' use of health care services to include historical, cultural, and sociopolitical contexts, the language we use and the interventions we devise seek only to change individuals' attitudes and behaviors rather than alter the conditions that deter clients from receiving adequate health care. Moreover, research tells us that individual behavior changes do not lead to significant reductions in overall morbidity and mortality in the absence of basic social, economic, and political changes (Freudenburg, 1984–85; Milio, 1986).

To meaningfully integrate equitable access to health care as a valued research and practice goal, nursing needs to move beyond conceptualizing at the individual level and instead theoretically frame access in its broadest sociopolitical context. Such is the objective of this paper. By critically exploring the concept of health care access in its broadest sense, describing the experiences and consequences of differential access, and providing rationale for the significance of this concept, the author lays the theoretical groundwork for more effective investigatory and practical action to assure equitable access. The purposes of this paper are to: provide a conceptual definition of equitable access, illustrate the theoretical dimensions of health care access in the U.S. through a synthesis of literatures, offer a critique of the status quo, and suggest implications for nursing research and practice.

CONCEPTUAL DEFINITION OF EQUITABLE ACCESS

The contention has been made that equitable access has never been defined in a rigorous fashion (Muurinen & Le Grand, 1985). If nurses are to ensure that practices and policies facilitate accessibility for all clients, a clear conceptualization of equitable access is needed. What is offered here is a definition of equitable access that incorporates dimensions of cost, geographic distribution, and quality. Economic and regional disenfranchisement from health services clearly compromises availability of preventive care and early detection and treatment of illness, drastically increasing morbidity and mortality. As well, health care encounters characterized by poor quality of care or negatively perceived interactions with health care providers perniciously affect health status and limit the field of health care options. In order for health care to be fully accessible it must be affordable, reasonably close by, and of sufficient quality, appropriateness, and sensitivity to encourage clients to continue to seek health care when they need it.

Equitable access to health care is defined by the following conditions: (1) relative costs of health care are experienced equally across all groups; (2) health care availability is based on the health needs and geographic distribution of the population rather than on the distribution of wealth; (3) health care encounters are of equal quality and comprehensiveness across all groups; and (4) health care interactions are positively perceived by all groups of clients so that continuing utilization of health care systems is facilitated.

DIMENSIONS OF EQUITABLE ACCESS

Economic and Geographic Accessibility

The first two conditions of equitable access address economic and geographic factors. Equitability of access means that all people face the same relative economic burden for health care costs and that the distribution of health care services is based on actual health circumstances of communities rather than on the socioeconomic status of individual clients. The concept of equitable access defines availability of health care as a matter of social responsibility rather than as a profit-making venture.

The capitalist organization of the current U.S. health care system encourages the structuring of health facilities as commercial enterprises (Waitzkin, 1983). This corporate fashioning forecloses crucial opportunities for care to uninsured persons and to many clients with conditions requiring extensive biomedical interventions, such as people with cancer or HIV illness. With the trend toward closure of public hospitals, providing services to these groups does not yield sufficient revenues to cover costs in privately owned for-profit facilities, health maintenance organizations, and preferred provider organizations, all of which reward the minimization of services.

According to MacPherson (1989), "the fundamental problem for nurses remains the contradiction between their mission to care for people and the profit orientation of a health care system that systematically curtails their opportunities to deliver nursing care" (p. 37). The increasing numbers of nurses employed in triage roles, whether by health care facilities, governments, or the insurance industry, is further evidence of this conflict between caregiving and gatekeeping in nursing. Although most people in the United States believe that everyone is entitled to health care and that withholding of health services is somehow immoral, one critic comments that, "given the present state of public health in the nation, rationing is both politically unspeakable and a daily reality. What occurs ... in public hospitals and clinics across the country, isn't rationing by rule but an invisible rationing carried out by nurses and doctors. They are constantly obliged by constraints of time and space and staff—constraints built into an underfunded system—to decide whom to help and whom not to help, just as on a battlefield" (Kirp, 1990, p. 306).

The relative costs of services, the travel to health care facilities, and the time and wages lost should be the same for all consumers. This premise suggests that clients with more intensive health care use, those living greater distances from health facilities, workers who stand to lose wages while ill, and those caring for dependent children, disabled persons, or elderly parents who must compensate others to fulfill these responsibilities when they are ill or injured, should pay less for health care services and be provided benefits to offset their losses (Muurinen & Le Grand, 1985). This notion stands in stark contrast to the current system which grants the "benefit" of health care according to the wage one earns and the capricious whims of one's insurance company.

Realities. The economic conditions requisite for equitable access do not exist in the United States. Ever larger segments of the U.S. population cannot obtain health care because of financial constraints (Aday, Andersen, & Fleming, 1980; Davis & Rowland, 1986; Dutton, 1978; Zambrana, 1987). At least 35 million Americans are without any health insurance coverage, having neither private policies nor public funding such as Medicaid (Davis & Rowland, 1986; Mitchell, Krueger, & Moody, 1990; Robert Wood Johnson Foundation, 1987). This figure indicates that 17% of the total U.S. population lacks coverage of any sort for health care costs, not because they choose to be unprotected, but because they cannot afford or are deemed ineligible for health care coverage (Bazzoli, 1986; Sulvetta & Swartz, 1986). An additional 17% are underinsured, which means that, because of gaps in coverage or cost-sharing requirements in their insurance policies, they risk an overwhelming financial burden should they become ill or injured (Farley, 1985).

Who suffers as a result of the way things are? Women, the poor, ethnic/racial minorities, and rural dwellers are disproportionately uninsured (Davis & Rowland,

1986; Meyer & Lewin, 1986; Trevino & Moss, 1984). Because they have no health insurance, they receive 50% less ambulatory health care and 90% fewer hospital services than insured persons (Davis & Rowland, 1983). Without the ability to pay for health services they are unable to obtain preventive care or early detection and treatment of illness and injury, the consequence of which is deteriorating health status (Muller, 1986b; Tallon & Block, 1987). Many are faced with unsurmountable health care bills if they do pursue services; others find that they are turned away from hospitals, even in times of emergency. Overcrowded, understaffed public hospitals often provide the only available care for the uninsured, but are, in fact, geographically accessible to only a fraction of those who need them (Schlesinger, 1987; Sloan, Valvona, & Mullner, 1986). These facts call into question nursing theories and practices that are predicated on individual choice and responsibility for seeking needed health services.

History. What historical trends have created the economic and political environment where such unequal access to health care is tolerated? The erosion of financial access can be attributed to several socioeconomic patterns over the past two decades, including: increased austerity applied to human services in the national budget, restricted public program eligibility, changes in employment, and unregulated growth of the insurance industry (Muller, 1986a; Tallon & Block, 1987).

Medicaid is not available to large segments of the population it was originally intended to serve. As a result of reduced federal support and increasing eligibility restrictions, today less than 50% of those who live below the poverty level are covered by Medicaid (Davis et al., 1987; Orr & Miller, 1981; U.S. Department of Health and Human Services, 1983; Walden, Wilensky, & Kaspar, 1985). The working poor and their families have largely been eliminated from Medicaid coverage (Cohen, 1990). Children have been a particularly vulnerable population in the midst of these changes. They represent 36% of the nation's 35 million uninsured individuals (U.S. Bureau of the Census, 1986b).

Employment trends, employer cost-containment strategies, and the weakening of the labor movement in this country over the past two decades are also major forces which have negatively affected health care access (Gimenez, 1989; Gordon-Bradshaw, 1987; Navarro, 1989). The decline of manufacturing and the tremendous growth of the service sector have reduced overall health insurance coverage because employers in nonunionized service industries do not ordinarily provide such benefits. Changing employment patterns including transitions in the labor force from union to nonunion, from full time to part time, and from high to low wages, have had a tremendous impact on the breadth of the population insured and the depth of benefits covered (Renner & Navarro, 1989). The 1980s also saw extensive reductions in employer responsibility for health care costs in more stable industries, through increased deductibles, major copayments, escalating employee contributions for dependent coverage, and the defunding of retiree health benefits (Greenhouse, 1986).

One author calls these employment trends "the immiseration of the working class" (Gimenez, 1989). Growing poverty within the working class is related to: higher rates of unemployment, the lowering of the average price of labor, union busting, right-to-work laws, cuts in benefits, stagnation of the minimum wage despite inflation, and the relocation of U.S. manufacturing to international sites where cheaper sources of labor are exploited (Gimenez, 1989; Gordon-Bradshaw, 1987).

Women's experiences are a case in point. Women are less likely to have the economic ability to pay for needed health care. They earn 65% of the wages earned by men in comparable jobs, a pattern that has persisted for 50 years (Ehrenberg & Smith, 1985; Estes, Gerard, & Clarke, 1984; Feldberg, 1984; Kelly & Bayes, 1988; O'Neill & Brown, 1981, U.S. Department of Labor, 1980). They are more likely to hold part-time jobs. Only 16% of part-time workers are enrolled in group health plans at work, while 72% of full-time workers enjoy such coverage (U.S. Bureau of the Census, 1986a). Despite dramatic increases in the female labor force, women are segregated into low-paying jobs where health insurance coverage and other benefits are less likely to be offered (Gimenez, 1989; Minkler & Stone, 1985; Smith, 1984; Wilson, 1987). Clerical, retail, and service work, categories of labor where women cluster are the fastest growing occupations, but they are also the occupations that have suffered the most extensive reductions in employer responsibility for health care costs (Tallon & Block, 1987).

Why do employment trends have such direct ramifications for health care access in this country? The United States is the only major industrialized nation whose health benefits coverage depends on job-related contributions; 85% of private health insurance coverage is employment based (Renner & Navarro, 1989). Health insurance coverage varies with the employment situation and is far from uniformly available. In fact, over three-quarters of the uninsured population is made up of employed persons and their dependents. Forty percent of uninsured adults work full time (Monheit, Hagan, Berk, & Farley, 1985). Aside from South Africa, the U.S. is the only industrialized nation that does not have a comprehensive and universal national health program.

A third major trend that diminishes access is the snowballing power of the insurance industry. Insurance companies increasingly refuse insurance coverage to particular types of workers, redlining entire job categories (Freudenheim, 1990). A wide variety of occupations have been declared ineligible for health insurance coverage by major insurers based on their profit-and-loss experiences with: service industries such as laundries, beauty salons, service stations, hotels, restaurants; hazardous and seasonal industries such as oil drilling, mining, logging, and fishing; and health care professions whose members are "highly aware of health care needs and thus tend to have a high rate of utilization" (p. 2).

Insurance companies also control their costs by actuarially limiting risks related to particular diagnoses such as AIDS, cancer, and other chronic illnesses, refusing coverage to individuals at risk for or suffering from these conditions. In many states, insurance companies can legally cancel the policies of clients who become ill (Garrison, 1990a). If people have shown a propensity to use health care for what are considered minor problems, they can also be rejected. Thus, many people find they cannot purchase policies at any price. Some insurers have gone so far as to reject all insurance applicants from San Francisco, which has the nation's largest AIDS caseload, and to deny health insurance to males who have jobs stereotypically associated with gay men (Lambert, 1989). As one author suggests, "Americans are increasingly slipping into ever-widening gaps in health coverage as the insurance industry changes its policies to insulate itself against rising medical costs" (Garrison, 1990b, p. 14).

There are other unregulated operations within the private insurance system that adversely affect access. Coverage often does not extend to conditions insurers declare are "preexisting." More and more insurers will not pay for state-of-the-art treatments, construing them as experimental. Premiums for smaller group plans can soar when one member gets ill or injured. So if a worker or his/her dependent experiences a serious health problem, the employer must either exclude that worker from insurance coverage or pass along higher premium rates to all the employees and risk losing insurance coverage for everyone.

Current U.S. laws do not protect individuals, groups, or communities from the health consequences of decreasing assistance program eligibility, decreasing employer accountability for health care coverage, or unregulated practices of insurance companies. Current emphases in nursing research do not target these problems of access. Current nursing practice, for the most part, is so tied to the socioeconomic agenda of corporate health care institutions that nurses feel powerless to impact access. To whom can health care consumers turn? Are we ignoring a fundamental disciplinary mandate? Clearly, practicing nurses have been enlisted in the "battle to contain health care costs," but have not had theoretical or tangible ethical support to advocate for consumers against cost-containment policies that negatively affect the availability and quality of health care. Nurses' unofficial assistance in the silent "rationing" of health care creates a moral and philosophical discord so intense that it is probably a major factor in the distress and disappointment experienced by so many practicing nurses who exit from the profession.

Qualitative and Interactional Accessibility

For health care to be accessible, it must not only be economically attainable and geographically at hand, but also qualitatively appropriate and nondiscriminatory. Health care encounters characterized by poor quality of care or negatively perceived interactions with health care providers can impair health status and limit the field of health care options. How can consumers feel free to seek health care if they believe they were inadequately treated or were oppressed in previous health care encounters?

Substantial differences in quality of health care across client groups have been documented (Chesney, Chavira, Hall, & Gary, 1982; Hayward, Shapiro, Freeman, & Corey, 1988; Muller, 1986a; Zambrana, 1987). This differential quality of care has taken the form of excessive waiting periods (Dutton, 1978; Finnerty, Mattie, & Finnerty, 1973), less thorough diagnostic evaluations (Armitage, Schneiderman, & Bass, 1979), withholding of indicated treatments (Fisher, 1984; Roth, 1986), and inappropriate and degrading interventions (Corea, 1985; Hurst & Zambrana, 1980; Scully, 1980; Shaw, 1974; Stevens & Hall, 1988). Investigations about health care interactions demonstrate that clinical decisions are made, not on the neutral grounds of health assessment alone, but with social criteria in mind (Fisher & Todd, 1983; Mishler, 1984; Wallen, Waitzkin, & Stoeckle, 1979). The operation of health care providers' unexamined prejudices and ethnocentrism is particularly apparent in health care interactions with women, persons of color, persons of low income, immigrants (especially those who do not speak English), gays, and lesbians (Anderson, 1985; Cartwright & O'Brien, 1976; Pendelton & Bochner, 1980; Todd, 1989; Townsend & Davidson, 1982; Waitzkin & Waterman, 1974). These clients are more likely to encounter treatment that does not fit their culture and life circumstances, and they are prone to receive stereotyped reactions and misdiagnoses because of qualitatively insensitive diagnostic procedures (Cochran & Mays, 1988; Cornely, 1976; Gibson, 1983; Hagebak & Hagebak, 1980; Jackson, 1977; Martin & Henry, 1989; Portillo, 1987; Quesada & Heller, 1977; Tripp-Reimer, 1982). They are more likely to be ignored, scolded, patronized, categorized as "difficult" patients, subjected to sexist and racist remarks, and provided fewer explanations of the health care they are receiving (Fisher & Groce, 1985; Jonas, 1974; La Fargue; 1972; Roth, 1975, 1986).

Lesbians' health care experiences exemplify these theoretical components of access (Stevens, 1992). Several investigations (Glascock, 1981; Johnson, Guenther, Laube, & Keetel, 1981; Paroski, 1987; Smith, Johnson, & Guenther, 1985; Stevens & Hall, 1988; Zeidenstein, 1990) suggest that lesbian clients frequently encounter hostile and discriminatory reactions from health care providers. Ostracism, invasive questioning, rough physical handling, derogatory comments, breaches of confidentiality, shock, embarrassment, unfriendliness, pity, condescension, and fear are among the reactions that surface in the provision of health care to this group of consumers. Some lesbians believe that health care providers' knowledge of their lesbianism could result in physical endangerment, infliction of pain, withdrawal of concern or neglect should providers harbor negative moral judgments about lesbians. Survey evidence indicates that their fears are legitimate (Harvey, Carr, & Bernheine, 1989; Levy, 1978; Mathews, Booth, Turner, & Kessler, 1986; Randall, 1989; White, 1979; Young, 1988). Significant numbers of physicians and nurses still consider lesbianism a pathological condition, make attributions of immorality, perversion, and danger to lesbian women, are uncomfortable providing care for lesbian clients, and regularly refuse service to them.

Lesbian clients' access is thus compromised. As a result of their negative experiences in health care encounters, many lesbian women hesitate to use health care systems and delay seeking treatment.

The evidence strongly suggests that nursing inquiry and practice geared toward improving access to health services must address race, gender, class, culture, and sexual orientation, acknowledging the role discriminatory behaviors can play in diminishing the availability of health care to large segments of the population. Nursing cannot insulate itself from the social conflicts and inequities that are faced by specific aggregates of consumers we serve.

CONSEQUENCES OF INEQUITABLE ACCESS

Limited access to affordable, high-quality, nondiscriminatory health care results in delay in seeking care, diagnosis and treatment in later stages of illness, and poorer prognosis (Gordon-Bradshaw, 1987). In the United States the most consistent pattern in the distribution of mortality and morbidity is their association with poverty. Death and disease rates vary inversely with social class (Kaplan, Haan, Syme, Minkler, & Winkleby, 1987; Kitagawa & Hauser, 1973; Minkler, 1989; Syme & Berkman, 1986). A disproportionate number of women and ethnic/racial minority people live in low-income households (Gimenez, 1989; Schlesinger, 1987). Their increased vulnerability to illness is significantly related to inequities in access to health care systems and differential quality of health care (Heckler, 1986; Makuc, Freid, & Kleinman, 1989; Manton, Patrick, & Johnson, 1987; U.S. Department of Health and Human Services, 1985). For instance, rates of death due to preventable and manageable conditions are 77% higher for African Americans than for Euro-Americans and are associated with poor access to existing medical, public health, and preventive services (Woolhandler et al., 1985).

Inequity in the availability of health services reinforces broader social disparities related to health status, such as inadequate income, poor nutrition, substandard housing, and unsafe occupations and neighborhoods (Davis, Gold, & Makuc, 1981). Improvements in access to and quality of health care for ethnic/racial minorities, poor and working class persons, sexual minorities, women, and children must therefore be accompanied by elimination of broader economic and social inequalities to achieve any real improvement in the health of individuals and communities (Miller, 1987).

The United States as a society seems to be increasingly tolerant of levels of poverty, denigration of women, homophobia, and racism that keep a growing number of people unhealthy, powerless, and without equal access to the resources needed for a full and healthy life. It strains the image of the United States as a just and humane society when significant portions of the population do not have ready access to health care, when profits are valued over people, and when individual clients are not accorded dignity and respect in health care encounters.

19

CONCLUSION

U.S. nursing is long overdue for action to stem the spiraling decline in access to health care. If we, as a scholarly and practice discipline, coalesce around the issue of equitable access to health care, making it a priority in our research, theory development, and clinical practice, we can change the tide. Nursing is the largest aggregate of health care providers. No other group is in a more strategic position to document and criticize the structural, interactional, and ideological circumstances that impede clients' access to and positive experience of health care. We have the knowledge, skills, and potential collective strength to be the architects of a radically new structure of health care delivery in this country, one that makes high-quality, nondiscriminatory health care universally available to everyone who lives in the United States.

We need nursing investigations that: (1) document the full range of aggregates' economic, geographic, qualitative, and interactional access to health care services; (2) explore the meanings and consequences of inequitable access in the lives of various groups of consumers; (3) analyze the economic, cultural, political, and social conditions that hamper access; (4) identify circumstances that facilitate access; and (5) point to nursing actions that will ensure equitable access. Nursing research is a political tool to be employed in arguing for structural change and in designing new programs, resources, and policies.

By constructing nursing theory that addresses real problems of access, rather than presuming ideal conditions for access to care, nursing scholars can lessen the theory-practice gap and provide a relevant basis for intervention. Any time we speak theoretically of health, health-promoting environments, or nursing therapeutics, we must be asking, "Who has access?"

In the practice arena, the key is collective action. As we analyze access to health care in its broadest social, economic, and political frame, we must also plan and implement interventions on this larger scale. We can join with other nurses and with consumers in local areas to identify practices and policies that limit accessibility. Then we can, as a group, place pressure on health care institutions, insurance companies, and governments to make changes. This means getting together with coworkers in collective bargaining units or in more informal collegial associations and meeting with clients, their significant others, and members of their communities to explore problems of access. We can utilize our nursing organizations, convincing them to prioritize equitable access. In coalition with consumer groups we can critique the current status of health care access and explore future options for universally accessible, comprehensive state and national health programs.

If we enlarge our conception of health care access and become knowledgeable about differential quality of care, geographic barriers, and economic exclusion of client groups, nurses can have a more articulate, powerful voice in saying who gets care. We will be able to: (1) avoid unwitting complicity in bureaucratic maneuvers that "ration" health care to selected populations; (2) reject ideologies that point to the "nursing shortage" as a rationale for inadequate access and poor quality care; and (3) interpret more accurately the constraints our clients contend with in obtaining health care. It is time for nurses to criticize the status quo rather than continue to focus all our energies on "working within the system," if indeed the present means of health care delivery can be called a "system." If we value what we do as nurses, the care we provide, then we have to be concerned about who gets that care.

REFERENCES

Aday, L. A., Andersen, R., & Fleming, G. V. (1980). *Health care in the U.S.: Equitable for whom?* Beverly Hills, CA: Sage.

American Nurses Association. (1980). *Nursing: A social-policy statement.* (Publ. No. NP-30). Kansas City, MO: American Nurses Association.

American Nurses Association Cabinet on Nursing Research. (1985). *Directions for nursing research: Toward the twenty-first century.* Kansas, City, MO: American Nurses Association.

Anderson, J. M. (1985). Perspectives on the health of immigrant women: A feminist analysis. *Advances in Nursing Science, 8*(1), 61–76.

Armitage, K. J., Schneiderman, L. J., & Bass, R. A. (1979). Response of physicians to medical complaints in men and women. *Journal of the American Medical Association, 241*(20), 2186–2187.

Bazzoli, G. J. (1986). Health care for the indigent: Overview of critical issues. *Health Services Research, 21*, 352–393.

Benner, P., & Wrubel, J. (1988). *The primacy of caring.* Menlo Park, CA: Addison-Wesley.

Butterfield, P. G. (1990). Thinking upstream: Nurturing a conceptual understanding of the societal context of health behavior. *Advances in Nursing Science, 12*(2), 1–8.

Cartwright, A., & O'Brien, M. C. (1976). Social class variation in health care. *The Sociology of the National Health Service: Sociological Review Monograph, 22*, 77–98.

Chesney, A. P., Chavira, J. A., Hall, R. P., & Gary, H. E. (1982). Barriers to medical care of Mexican-Americans: The role of social class, acculturation, and social isolation. *Medical Care, 20*(9), 883–891.

Cochran, S. D., & Mays, V. M. (1988). Disclosure of sexual preference to physicians by Black lesbian and bisexual women. *Western Journal of Medicine, 149*(5), 616–619.

Cohen, S. S. (1990). The politics of Medicaid: 1980–1989. *Nursing Outlook, 38*(5), 229–233.

Corea, G. (1985). *The hidden malpractice: How American medicine mistreats women.* New York: Harper & Row.

Cornely, P. B. (1976). Racism: The ever present hidden barrier to health in our society. *American Journal of Public Health, 66*, 246–247.

Davis, G. C. (1988). Nursing values and health care policy. *Nursing Outlook, 36*(6), 289–292.

Davis, K., Gold, M., & Makuc, D. (1981). Access to health care for the poor: Does the gap remain? *Annual Review of Public Health, 2*, 159–182.

Davis, K., Lillie-Blanton, M., Lyons, B., Mullan, F., Powe, N., & Rowland, D. (1987). Health care for Black Americans: The public sector role. *The Milbank Quarterly, 65*(1), 213–247.

Davis, K., & Rowland, D. (1986). Uninsured and underserved: Inequities in health care in the United States. In P. Conrad & R. Kern (Eds.), *The sociology of health and illness: Critical perspectives* (pp. 250–266). New York: St. Martin's Press.

Davis, K., & Rowland, D. (1983). Uninsured and underserved: Inequities in health care in the United States. *The Milbank Memorial Fund Quarterly, 61*(2), 160–166.

Dimond, M. (1989). Health care and the aging population. *Nursing Outlook, 37*(2), 76–77.

Dutton, D. B. (1978). Explaining the low use of health services by the poor: Costs, attitudes, or delivery systems? *American Sociological Review, 43,* 348–368.

Ehrenberg, R. G., & Smith, R. S. (1985). *Modern labor economics: Theory and public policy.* Glenview, IL: Scott, Foresman.

Estes, C. L., Gerard, L., & Clarke, A. (1984). Women and the economics of aging. *International Journal of Health Services, 14*(1), 55–68.

Farley, P. (1985). Who are the uninsured? *The Milbank Memorial Fund Quarterly, 63*(3), 477.

Feldberg, R. L. (1984). Comparable worth: Toward theory and practice in the United States. *Signs: Journal of Women in Culture and Society, 10*(2), 311–328.

Finnerty, F. A., Mattie, E. C., & Finnerty, F. A. (1973). Hypertension in the inner city: I. Analysis of clinic dropouts. *Circulation, 47,* 73–78.

Fisher, S. (1984). Doctor-patient communication: A social and micro-political performance. *Sociology of Health and Illness, 6*(1), 1–29.

Fisher, S., & Groce, S. B. (1985). Doctor-patient negotiation of cultural assumptions. *Sociology of Health and Illness, 7*(3), 342–374.

Fisher, S., & Todd, A. D. (Eds.) (1983). *The social organization of doctor-patient communication.* Washington, DC: Center for Applied Linguistics.

Freudenberg, N. (1984–85). Training health educators for social change. *International Quarterly of Community Health Education, 5*(1), 37–52.

Freudenheim, M. (1990, February 6). Many health insurers blacklisting several types of workers. *San Francisco Chronicle,* p. 2.

Funkhouser, S. W., & Moser, D. K. (1990). Is health care racist? *Advances in Nursing Science, 12*(2), 47–55.

Garrison, J. (1990a, October 21). Insurance firm abandons clients: Sick people lost health coverage to boost profits. *San Francisco Examiner,* pp. 1, 20.

Garrison, J. (1990b, October 7). Policy changes exclude the sick, protect the few. *San Francisco Examiner,* pp.1, 14–15.

Gibson, G. (1983). Hispanic women: Stress and mental health issues. *Women and Therapy, 2*(2–3), 113–133.

Gimenez, M. E. (1989). The feminization of poverty: Myth or reality? *International Journal of Health Services, 19*(1), 45–61.

Glascock, E. L. (1981, November). *Access to the traditional health care system by non-traditional women: Perceptions of a cultural interaction.* Paper presented at American Public Health Association Annual Meeting, Los Angeles.

Gordon-Bradshaw, R. H. (1987). A social essay on special issues facing poor women of color. *Women & Health, 12*(3–4), 243–259.

Greenhouse, S. (1986, August 24). Health plans are feeling a little peaked. *The New York Times,* p. E5.

Hagebak, J. E., & Hagebak, B. R. (1980). Serving the mental health needs of the elderly: The case for removing barriers and improving service integration. *Community Mental Health Journal, 16,* 263–272.

Hall, J. M., & Stevens, P. E. (1991). The nursing shortage in the context of national health care. *Nursing Outlook, 39*(2), 69–72.

Harrington, C. A. (1988). A national health care program: Has its time come? *Nursing Outlook, 36*(5), 214–216, 255.

Harrington, C. A. (1990). Policy options for a national health care plan. *Nursing Outlook, 38*(5), 223–228.

Harvey, S. M., Carr, C., & Bernheine, S. (1989). Lesbian mothers: Health care experiences. *Journal of Nurse-Midwifery, 34*(3), 115–119.

Hayward, R. A., Shapiro, M. F., Freeman, H. E., & Corey, C. R. (1988). Inequities in health services among insured Americans. *New England Journal of Medicine, 318,* 1507–1512.

Heckler, M. M. (1986). *Report of the secretary's task force on Black and minority health.* Washington, DC: U.S. Department of Health and Human Services.

Hodnicki, D. R. (1990). Homelessness: Health-care implications. *Journal of Community Health Nursing, 7*(2), 59–67.

Hurst, M., & Zambrana, R. E. (1980). The health careers of urban women: A study in East Harlem. *Signs: Journal of Women in Culture and Society, 5*(3), S112–S126.

Jackson, R. (1977). Barriers to health care delivery. *Washington State Journal of Nursing, 49*(1), 11–15.

Johnson, S. R., Guenther, S. M., Laube, D. W., Keettel, W. C. (1981). Factors influencing lesbian gynecological care: A preliminary study. *American Journal of Obstetrics and Gynecology, 140*(1), 20–28.

Jonas, S. (1974). Health, health care and racism. *Hospitals, 48*(4), 72–75.

Kaplan, G. A., Haan, M., Syme, S. L., Minkler, M., & Winkleby, M. (1987). Socioeconomic status and health. *American Journal of Epidemiology, 125,* 989–998.

Kelly, R. M., & Bayes, J. (Eds.). (1988). *Comparable worth, pay equity, and public policy.* Westport, CT: Greenwood Press.

Kidder, L. H., & Fine, M. (1986). Making sense of injustice. In E. Seidman & J. Rappaport (Eds.), *Redefining social problems* (pp. 49–64). New York: Plenum Press.

Kirp, D. L. (1990). Rationing life and death. *The Nation, 250*(9), 306–308.

Kitagawa, E. M., & Hauser, P. M. (1973). *Differential mortality in the U.S.: A study in socioeconomic epidemiology.* Cambridge, MA: Harvard University Press.

La Fargue, J. P. (1972). Role of prejudice in rejection of health care. *Nursing Research, 21*(1), 53–58.

Lambert, B. (1989, August 7). Insurance limits growing to curb AIDS coverage. *The New York Times,* pp. 1, 9.

Leininger, M. M. (1988). *Caring: An essential human need.* Detroit: Wayne State University.

Levy, T. (1978). *The lesbian: As perceived by mental health workers.* Unpublished doctoral dissertation, California School of Professional Psychology, San Diego.

MacPherson, K. I. (1989). A new perspective on nursing and caring in a corporate context. *Advances in Nursing Science, 11*(4), 32–39.

MacPherson, K. I. (1987). Health policy, values and nursing. *Advances in Nursing Science, 9*(3), 1–11.

Makuc, D. M., Freid, V. M., & Kleinman, J. C. (1989). National trends in the use of preventive health care by women. *American Journal of Public Health, 79*(1), 21–26.

Manton, K. G., Patrick, C. H., & Johnson, K. W. (1987). Health differentials between Blacks and whites: Recent trends in mortality and morbidity. *The Milbank Quarterly, 65*(1), 129–199.

Martin, M. E., & Henry, M. (1989). Cultural relativity and poverty. *Public Health Nursing, 6*(1), 28–34.

Mathews, W. C., Booth, M. W., Turner, J. D., & Kessler, L. (1986). Physicians' attitudes toward homosexuality: Survey of a California county medical society. *Western Journal of Medicine, 144*(1), 106–110.

Meyer, J. A., & Lewin, M. E. (1986). Poverty and social welfare: An agenda for change. *Inquiry, 23*, 122–133.

Milio, N. (1986). *Promoting health through public policy*. Ottawa, Ontario: Canadian Public Health Association.

Milio, N. (1988). The profitization of health promotion. *International Journal of Health Services, 18*(4), 573–585.

Miller, S. M. (1987). Race in the health of America. *The Milbank Memorial Fund Quarterly, 65*(2), 500–531.

Minkler, M. (1989). Health education, health promotion and the open society: An historical perspective. *Health Education Quarterly, 16*(1), 17–30.

Minkler, M., & Stone, R. (1985). The feminization of poverty and older women. *Gerontologist, 25*(4), 351–357.

Mishler, E. G. (1984). *The discourse of medicine*. Norwood, NJ: Ablex.

Mitchell, P. H., Krueger, J. C., & Moody, L. E. (1990). The crisis of the health care nonsystem. *Nursing Outlook, 38*(5), 214–217.

Moccia, P. (1988). At the faultline: Social activism and caring. *Nursing Outlook, 36*(1), 30–33.

Moccia, P., & Mason, D. J. (1986). Poverty trends: Implications for nursing. *Nursing Outlook, 34*(1), 20–24.

Monheit, A., Hagan, M., Berk, M., & Farley, P. (1985). The employed uninsured and the role of social policy. *Inquiry, 22*, 349.

Muller, C. (1986a). Review of twenty years of research on medical care utilization. *Health Services Research, 21*(2), 129–144.

Muller, C. (1986b). Women and men: Quality and equality in health care. *Social Policy, 17*(1), 39–45.

Muurinen, J. M., & Le Grand, J. (1985). The economic analysis of inequalities in health. *Social Science and Medicine, 20*(10), 1029–1035.

Navarro, V. (1989). Why some countries have national health insurance, others have national health services, and the U.S. has neither. *Social Science and Medicine, 28*(9), 887–898.

O'Neill, J., & Brown, R. (1981). *Women and the labor market: A survey of issues and policies in the U.S.* Washington, DC: Urban Institute.

Orr, S. T., & Miller, C. A. (1981). Utilization of health services by poor children since the advent of Medicaid. *Medical Care, 19*(6), 583–590.

Paroski, P. A. (1987). Health care delivery and the concerns of gay and lesbian adolescents. *Journal of Adolescent Health Care, 8*(2), 188–192.

Paterson, J. G., & Zderad, L. T. (1976). *Humanistic nursing*. New York: John Wiley & Sons.

Pendelton, D., & Bochner, S. (1980). The communication of medical information in general practice consultations as a function of patients' social class. *Social Science and Medicine, 14A*, 669–673.

Portillo, C. T. (1987). Poverty, self-concept, and health: Experience of Latinas. *Women & Health, 12*(3–4), 229–242.

Quesada, G. M., & Heller, P. L. (1977). Sociocultural barriers to medical care among Mexican Americans in Texas. *Medical Care, 15*(5), 93–101.

Randall, C. E. (1989). Lesbian phobia among BSN educators: A survey. *Journal of Nursing Education, 28*(7), 302–306.

Renner, C., & Navarro, V. (1989). Why is our population of uninsured and underinsured persons growing? The consequences of the "deindustrialization" of America. *Annual Review of Public Health, 10*, 85–94.

Robert Wood Johnson Foundation. (1987). *Access to health care in the United States: Results of a 1986 survey*. Special Report no. 2. Princeton, NJ: Princeton University.

Rooks, J. P. (1990). Let's admit we ration health care—then set priorities. *American Journal of Nursing, 90*(6), 39–43.

Ross, J. W. (1989). AIDS, rationing of care, and ethics. *Family and Community Health, 12*(2), 24–33.

Roth, J. A. (1986). Some contingencies of the moral evaluation and control of clientele: The case of the hospital emergency service. In P. Conrad & R. Kern (Eds.), *The sociology of health and illness: Critical perspectives* (pp. 322–333). New York: St. Martin's Press.

Roth, J. A. (1975). The treatment of the sick. In J. Kosa & I. K. Zola (Eds.), *Poverty and health: A sociological analysis* (pp. 274–302). Cambridge, MA: Harvard University Press.

Ryan, W. (1971). *Blaming the victim.* New York: Vintage.

Schlesinger, M. (1987). Paying the price: Medical care, minorities, and the newly competitive health care system. *The Milbank Quarterly, 65*(2), 270–296.

Scully, D. (1980). *Men who control women's health.* Boston: Houghton Mifflin.

Seidman, E., & Rappaport, J. (Eds.). (1986). *Redefining social problems.* New York: Plenum Press.

Shaw, N. S. (1974). *Forced labor: Maternity care in the U.S.* New York: Pergamon Press.

Sloan, F., Valvona, J., & Mullner, R. (1986). Identifying the issues: A statistical profile. In F. Sloan, J. Blumstein, & J. Perrin (Eds.), *Uncompensated hospital care: Rights and responsibilities* (pp. 19–24). Baltimore: Johns Hopkins University Press.

Smith, E. M., Johnson, S. R., & Guenther, S. M: (1985). Health care attitudes and experiences during gynecological care among lesbians and bisexuals. *American Journal of Public Health, 75*(9), 1085–1087.

Smith, J. (1984). The paradox of women's poverty: Wage-earning women and economic transformation. *Signs: Journal of Women in Culture and Society, 20*(2), 291–310.

Smith, J. P. (1990). The politics of American health care. *Journal of Advanced Nursing, 15*(4), 487–497.

Stevens, P. E. (1992). Lesbian health care research: A review of the literature from 1970 to 1990. *Health Care for Women International, 13*(2), 91–120.

Stevens, P. E., & Hall, J. M. (1988). Stigma, health beliefs and experiences with health care in lesbian women. *Image: Journal of Nursing Scholarship, 20*(2), 69–73.

Sulvetta, M., & Swartz, K. (1986). *The uninsured and uncompensated care: A chartbook.* Washington, DC: National Health Policy Forum.

Syme, S. L., & Berkman, L. F. (1986). Social class, susceptibility, and sickness. In P. Conrad & R. Kern (Eds.), *The sociology of health and illness: Critical perspectives* (pp. 28–34). New York: St. Martin's Press.

Tallon, J. R., & Block, R. (1987). Changing patterns of health insurance coverage: Special concerns for women. *Women and Health, 12*(3–4), 119–136.

Todd, A. D. (1989). *Intimate adversaries: Cultural conflict between doctors and women patients.* Philadelphia: University of Pennsylvania Press.

Townsend, P., & Davidson, P. (1982). *Inequalities in health.* London: Penguin.

Trevino, F. M., & Moss, A. J. (1984). *Health insurance for Hispanic, Black, and white Americans.* Vital and Health Statistics (Series 10. No. 148). Washington, DC: U. S. Public Health Service, National Center for Health Statistics. (DHHS Publication No. PHS 84-1576).

Tripp-Reimer, T. (1982). Barriers to health care: Variations in interpretation of Appalachian client behavior by Appalachian and non-Appalachian health professionals. *Western Journal of Nursing Research, 4*(2), 179–191.

U.S. Bureau of the Census. (1986a). Characteristics of households and persons receiving selected noncash benefits: 1984. *Current Population Report (Series P-60, No. 150).* Washington, DC: U.S. Government Printing Office.

U.S. Bureau of the Census. (1986b). Money, income, and poverty status of families and persons in the U.S.: 1986. *Current Population Report (Series P-60, No. 157)*. Washington, DC: U.S. Government Printing Office.

U.S. Department of Health and Human Services. (1985). *Black and minority health* (Report of the Secretary's Task Force, Executive Summary, Vol.I). Washington, DC: U.S. Department of Health and Human Services.

U.S. Department Of Health and Human Services. (1983). *The Medicare and Medicaid data book.* Baltimore: U.S. Department of Health and Human Services.

U.S. Department of Labor. (1980). *Facts on women workers.* Washington, DC: Office of Information Publications & Reports.

Waitzkin, H. (1983). *The second sickness: Contradictions of capitalistic health care.* New York: Free Press.

Waitzkin, H. B., & Waterman, B. (1974). *The exploitation of illness in capitalist society.* Indianapolis: Bobbs-Merrill.

Walden, D., Wilensky, G., & Kaspar, J. (1985). *Changes in health insurance status: Full year and part year coverage, data preview 21.* Rockville, MD: U.S. Department of Health and Human Services.

Wallen, J., Waitzkin, H., & Stoeckle, J. D. (1979). Physician stereotypes about female health and illness: A study of patient's sex and the information process during medical interviews. *Women and Health, 4,* 135–146.

Watson, J. (1985). *Nursing: The philosophy and science of caring.* Boulder, CO: Colorado Associated University Press.

White, T. A. (1979). Attitudes of psychiatric nurses toward same sex orientations. *Nursing Research, 28*(5), 276–281.

Williams, D. M. (1989). Political theory and individualistic health promotion. *Advances in Nursing Science, 12*(1), 14–25.

Wilson, J. B. (1987). Women and poverty: A demographic overview. *Women and Health, 12*(3–4), 21–40.

Woolhandler, S., Himmelstein, D. U., Silber, R., Bader, M., Harnly, M., & Jones, A. A. (1985). Medical care and mortality: Racial differences in preventable deaths. *International Journal of Health Services, 15*(1), 1–22.

Young, E. W. (1988). Nurses' attitudes toward homosexuality: Analysis of change in AIDS workshops. *Journal of Continuing Education in Nursing, 19*(1), 9–12.

Zambrana, R. E. (1987). A research agenda on issues affecting poor and minority women: A model for understanding their health needs. *Women and Health, 12*(3–4), 137–160.

Zeidenstein, L. (1990). Gynecological and childbearing needs of lesbians. *Journal of Nurse-Midwifery, 35*(1), 10–18.

Offprints. Requests for offprints should be sent to Patricia E. Stevens, R.N., Ph.D., 1612 Noriega Street, San Francisco, CA 94122.

2

Ethical Foundations in Nursing for Broad Health Care Access

Mila Ann Aroskar, R.N., Ed.D., F.A.A.N.

University of Minnesota

Stevens' article on health care access is a comprehensive discussion of an issue that is currently center stage on the national scene. Her article raises important questions about the centrality of this issue in the nursing community, specifically in practice, research, and theory. Stevens states in this article that nurses have not had ethical support to advocate for access to health care. Nurses do have ethical support and a moral mandate for such activity in the American Nurses Association's *Code for Nurses* (1976; 1985).

The *Code for Nurses* makes explicit nursing's goals and values, its moral obligations to patients and clients. One of the nurses' obligations is to work with other health professionals and citizens to promote efforts to meet the health needs of the public. More explicitly, the interpretive statements claim that nurses have obligations "*to promote equitable access to nursing and health care for all people*" and to actively participate in activities that ensure the availability and accessibility of high-quality health services to all persons with unmet health needs. These statements are unequivocal in support of an ethical obligation and mandate for nurses to be involved in health care access issues.

The first code approved by ANA in 1950 included the same broad obligation (Fowler, 1984). It says, in the spirit of the current code, that nurses should participate and share responsibility with others in promoting efforts to meet the public's health needs in local, state, national and international settings. Nursing has had this broad mandate, then, longer than the past decade. The mandate includes specific concerns for access to health care.

A bleak reality exists for nurses, nursing, and our proclaimed clients, according to Stevens. She signals a relative lack of action in significant parts of the nursing community with regard to this moral obligation. This moral obligation has existed for the last half of the 20th century in the code that is a public statement of what the profession considers to be its moral obligations and values. The *Code for Nurses* alone provides ethical support and a moral imperative for nurses to be involved in access to health care issues and related public policy. Yet, for the most part—with a few noteworthy exceptions—we continue to focus on issues of

27

individual patient care in nursing and hold a mindset that nurses who work in arenas of public policy and politics have "left" nursing.

The focus of nurses and other health care providers on individual care is not surprising. There are several possible explanations for this focus. They include: (1) the first obligation mentioned in the *Code* which emphasizes respectful care of individuals, (2) the individual focus of much advocacy literature in nursing, (3) the traditional medical ethic that requires doing everything possible for the individual patient, (4) society's emphasis on individualism and individual freedom of choice, and (5) the bioethics literature's emphasis, until recently, on individual autonomy and rights. Even the stated commitments of community and public health nursing to the health of communities and populations at risk and to education dealing with participation in the legislative process and policy development have not been an effective counterbalance to a focus on the individual in health care and in our society. Such realities do not serve as justification for a continuing lack of attention to access issues in nursing practice, research, and theory development.

A recent counterpoint to the focus on individual client care in nursing is *Nursing's Agenda for Health Care Reform* (American Nurses Association, 1991), endorsed by more than 50 nursing organizations. The Agenda is reflective of nursing's values and has profound implications for public policy development. It calls for immediate restructuring of health care in our country and proposes universal consumer access to a standard package of essential services to be delineated at the federal level. This document claims that "America's nurses have long supported our nation's efforts to create a health care system that assures access, quality, and services at affordable costs." The question still remains: How central is the issue of health care access to nurses in practice, research, and theory? My claim here is the existence of solid ethical support for nurses to work on access issues as a moral obligation in the *Code for Nurses*, in Stevens' concept of equitable access as a matter of social responsibility and nursing accountability to society, and in discussions of nursing and public policy in the nursing ethics literature (see, for example, Davis & Aroskar, 1991).

A major challenge to achieving some level of access to health care for all is the lack of a societal consensus on what constitutes justice. This is the case for an understanding of justice broadly and, more narrowly, for an understanding of what constitutes distributive justice in health care. Justice is foundational to this structure of society and to structures for delivery of nursing and health care services. We all may agree that the present lack of access to health care for millions in the world's wealthiest country is unjust. Agreement on what is unjust does not automatically tell us what justice should be. So, major conceptual challenges continue to exist in efforts to clarify what constitutes justice and how to construct a more just society in which everyone has assurance of access to health care when resources are finite.

A related and fundamental question for our society concerns the appropriate goals for health care. How should wellness and prevention be balanced with high-tech care in terms of allocating society's finite resources? Once society has identified its goals for health care, how should the benefits and burdens of health care be distributed to meet these goals? What is the morally justifiable basis for such a distribution? What should all Americans have access to in health care? If we cannot afford to provide everything available and medically appropriate for everyone, what services should be assured for everyone? I am concerned that these complex questions are difficult, if not impossible, to adequately answer without some consensus on what constitutes justice in our society.

Several ideas about distributive justice compete for attention in distribution of health care and other social goods and resources such as education. These ideas include contracts, individual needs, individual effort, societal contribution, ability to pay, merit, and equal shares. Different ideas about distributive justice and distribution of social goods, individually and in combination, are used in different contexts. Welfare payments are distributed on the basis of need, while jobs and promotions are distributed on the basis of achievement and merit (Beauchamp & Childress, 1989). In health care, we often invoke needs and rights as a basis for claims about access. Health care services in the U.S. today, however, are available primarily according to ability to pay. Clearly, this is not an ethically justifiable basis for access to health care. As individuals we have not chosen our genetic makeup that influences health status or the socioeconomic circumstances into which which we were born. On this basis, the President's Commission for the Study of Ethical Problems in Medicine and Biomedical and Behavioral Research, in a report on access, concluded that assuring equitable access to health care is a societal obligation (1983). Claims for such an ethical obligation in the *Code for Nurses* is congruent with this conclusion.

Largely unsuccessful efforts at cost containment in health care during the past two decades have re-focused attention on the fact that individual client care occurs in a socioeconomic context where the focus on autonomy of individual patients and providers should not be allowed to trump other values such as fair access to health care. In addition to the nursing documents already discussed, other non-nursing resources are available that provide further support for nursing action in practice, research, and theory development to influence who gets health care.

The report on access to health care by the President's Commission (1983) is an example of a resource that nursing should use in efforts to make health care access an "arena for nursing action" in practice, research, theory, and education. This commission was mandated by Congress in the late 1970s to examine ethical issues and problems in health care beyond the protection of human subjects in research. The commission no longer exists due primarily to political constraints. Carolyn Williams, Dean and Professor at the College of Nursing at the University of Kentucky, served as the only nurse member of the commission.

A second resource is the report of a University of Minnesota Center for Biomedical Ethics project exploring the moral foundations of our health care system (Priester, 1992). The major argument of this report is that current health care-reform efforts to deal with fundamental system problems are doomed to failure without an adequate framework of shared values to guide reform, to serve as a rallying point for building consensus about health care reform, and to evaluate proposals for reform. Ignoring or uncritically accepting the "old" values underlying health care since World War II, such as professional autonomy and consumer sovereignty in the health care market, contributes to the incremental, piecemeal, and reactive responses that characterize most current proposals for reform.

The "new"-values framework proposed in the University of Minnesota project report makes fair access to health care the priority value, reversing the traditional balance between autonomy and access. Fair access, quality, efficiency, respect for patients, and patient advocacy are viewed as essential values, that is, fundamental values for the health care system. Instrumental values that contribute to achieving and promoting the essential values include three community-oriented values that are missing from the current framework. The community values are added to provide balance for the excessive individualism that has prevailed in health care and in American society. These values are: social advocacy, personal responsibility, and social solidarity.

Social advocacy calls on health providers to actively advocate for the needs of underserved people and of our entire society. The value of personal responsibility requires that everyone share in the cost of health care, that clients use health care services appropriately, and that education is provided to inform and enable individuals to maintain and improve their health. Part of operationalizing this concept of personal responsibility includes the selection of efficient health care plans and providers. The value of social solidarity could be considered as the "glue" that fosters a recognition by all citizens of our social, political, and economic interdependence, as well as a perception of shared ownership. This value is viewed as helping to promote a health care system that holds the value of fair access preeminent. According to the report (Priester, 1992), adopting the value of social solidarity may be necessary in our social value system to shift U.S. health policy from the excessive emphasis on individualism. This value's framework is proposed to be the moral foundation of America's health care system and the guide for health care policy. These are only two examples of a wider literature on ethics, values, and access to health care.

In conclusion, nurses have ethical support for and a moral imperative to make access to health care an explicit arena for nursing action. No part of the nursing community is exempt from this endeavor—practice, research, theory development, and education. Taking this imperative seriously could provide an antidote for what Stevens describes as "nurses' unofficial assistance in the silent 'rationing' of health care [that] creates a moral and philosophical discord so intense that it is probably a major factor in the distress and disappointment experienced by so many practicing nurses who exit from the profession." Access to health care should be a central concern in nursing practice, research, and theory development. Stevens provides suggestions for ways to make this a reality in nursing for the benefit of nursing's clients.

REFERENCES

American Nurses Association. (1976, 1985). *Code for nurses with interpretive statements*. Kansas City, MO: Author.

American Nurses Association. (1991). *Nursing's agenda for health care reform*. (1991). Supplement to *The American Nurse*. Kansas City, MO: Author.

Beauchamp, T. L., & Childress, J. F. (1989). *Principles of biomedical ethics* (3rd ed.). New York: Oxford.

Davis, A. J., & Aroskar, M. A. (1991). *Ethical dilemmas and nursing practice* (3rd ed.). Norwalk, CT: Appleton & Lange.

Fowler, M. D. M. (1984). *Ethics and nursing, 1893–1984. The ideal of service, the reality of history*. Dissertation. Los Angeles: University of Southern California.

Priester, R. (1992, Spring). A values framework for health system reform. *Health Affairs, 11*, 84–107.

Offprints. Requests for offprints should be sent to Mila Ann Aroskar, R.N., Ed.D., F.A.A.N., University of Minnesota, Division of Health Services Administration, School of Public Health, Box 97, C309 Mayo Memorial Building, 420 Delaware Street, SE, Minneapolis, MN 55455.

3

A Nursing Policy Perspective

Virginia Trotter Betts, M.S.N., J. D., R.N.

Vanderbilt Institute for Public Policy Studies
American Nurses Association

The 1990s health policy debate reflects some consensus about the three key aspects of the health care dilemma: limited access, escalating costs, and questionable quality. As of mid-1992, there were no less than 38 proposals for health care reform circulating in the policy/politics circles of the nation. Most purport to have solutions for the nation to consider in building a new health care infrastructure.

On analysis, almost all of the plans have a commonality—the agreement that universal access for all citizens of the U.S. is a must. After all, the only *other* industrialized nation in the world without universal access is South Africa—a nation that few Americans would choose to emulate.

One plan that deserves and is receiving serious consideration as a health reform document is *Nursing's Agenda for Health Care Reform.* Developed by the American Nurses Association in collaboration with the National League for Nursing, the policy proposal has now been endorsed widely in the organized nursing community. It is *the* plan, representing a futuristic health agenda for over 55 nursing groups. Nursing's plan significantly addresses access to health care.

The access portion of the health policy problem is usually described as populations who are uninsured or underinsured. The uninsured are those who are apt to be locked out of the health delivery system because they have no "ticket" to guarantee payment for medical care in case of illness or injury. Recent estimates project that 34.6 million persons are in this category. Twenty million are workers and 8.4 million are children under the age of 18. Seventy-two percent of the uninsured have incomes above the federal poverty line, but income has a direct correlation with those who purchase individual insurance when no group policy is available. Only 1 in 40 employees remains uninsured when offered a group policy (Robert Wood Johnson Foundation, 1992).

The numbers of underinsured are a matter of continuing debate/definition. The underinsured include individuals who have some health coverage, but it is so limited as to be ineffective in the event of a variety of serious illnesses/injuries. The usual estimate is one equal to the number of uninsured but this appears to be significantly underestimated as it includes neither the Medicare or Medicaid

33

populations. More reliable data on the underinsured are expected in fall 1992 (Robert Wood Johnson Foundation, 1992).

Nursing's Agenda for Health Care Reform calls for the inclusion of all citizens and residents of the U.S. to be covered for a basic core of federally defined health care services provided through a public plan or private employer plans (American Nurses Association, 1991). While nursing's plan may be said to be basically a "pay or play" scheme, it really is more innovative in that the public plan will ultimately combine Medicare, Medicaid, and other public initiatives and will be attractive to individuals and small businesses as a cost-effective plan (large group rates) through which to purchase the basic benefit plan. Private plans will be altered to: (a) include all basic benefits and (b) eliminate current insurance industry efforts to "cream" off good risks and leave individuals with poor health histories without coverage at an affordable cost.

Access to health care, however, is more than just the ability to pay. Additionally, access is linked to the availability of providers and the acceptability to the consumer of the care provided. Most of the health reform plans before the public do not address these other important access variables. Most reforms assume that "fixing" the payment variables will assure access for all. Such reasoning disregards the tremendous difficulty in placing an appropriate mix of qualified providers in rural and inner-city areas and in identifying innovative care strategies needed by vulnerable populations which have increased risk by virtue of race, socioeconomic status, and/or special health needs.

Organized nursing's *Agenda for Health Care Reform* speaks to the tripartite causes of limited health care access while furthering the profession's longstanding commitment to health care as a right and not a privilege. In fact, two cornerstones of nursing's plan—(a) consumer choice and responsibility for selfcare with informed consent and (b) consumer access to a variety of qualified providers—go to the heart of the nonfinancial access problem (American Nurses Association, 1991).

Professional nurses have, as part of the code of ethics, an obligation to include the client in decision making and in advocating for client choices within the health care system (American Nurses Association, 1985). Clients of nurses have responded to this partnership with a positive view of the nurse and with active participation in health care regimes. For example, certified nurse midwives (CNMs) safely manage normal pregnancies as well as or better than physicians (Jacox, 1987). CNMs' care reflects fewer low-birth-weight babies and shorter inpatient post-delivery days. Patients of CNMs report greater satisfaction with care and highlight communication and the ability to be more self-determining during delivery (Jacox, 1987). Thus professional nurses and *Nursing's Agenda for Health Reform* consistently deal with questions of access as acceptability.

As for access as availability, professional nurses are the foot soldiers of the health delivery system. Nurses care for the poor, the disadvantaged, the chronically mentally and physically ill. Nurse practitioners (NPs) enhanced access to primary care dramatically during the 1970s. In 1980, 47.3% of NPs provided care in inner cities and 9.4% of NPs practiced in rural areas (Jacox, 1987). In 1991, an assessment of NPs in Oregon concluded that NPs were much more likely than physicians to locate in remote rural areas and to stay in practice in these areas (Office of Rural Health, 1991).

Professional nurses seek through policy and politics to be available to clients who need care. Significant barriers to the availability of advanced practice nurses in every state include restrictive scope of practice legislation and regulation and the limited reimbursement practices of both public and private insurers. *Nursing's Agenda for Health Care Reform* calls for an end to such artificial barriers that diminish access to nursing services and thus to primary care.

Certainly, as organized nursing moves forcefully into this era of the health reform debate, much more research as to nursing's costs, benefits, and outcomes is needed. Let us not overlook the dramatic importance of *Nursing's Agenda for Health Care Reform*, however, in putting forth a blueprint for nursing activism in policy, politics, research, and practice for years to come. *Access* is a significant strength of *Nursing's* proposal. All elements of access—affordability, availability, and acceptability—are markedly addressed by *Nursing's* plan and, in my view, by today's nursing leaders.

REFERENCES

American Nurses Association. (1985). *Code for nurses.* Kansas City: Author.

American Nurses Association. (1991). *Nursing's agenda for health reform.* Kansas City: Author.

Congress of the United States, Office of Technology Assessment. (1986, March). Health Technology, Case Study 37. *Nurse practitioners, physicians' assistants, and certified nurse midwives: A policy analysis.*

Jacox, A. (1987). The OTA report: A policy analysis. *Nursing Outlook, 35*(5), 262–267.

Office of Rural Health. (1991). *Nurse practitioners and physician assistants in Oregon.*

Robert Wood Johnson Foundation. (1992, March). *Updata, 3*(1).

Offprints. Requests for offprints should be sent to Virginia Trotter Betts, MSN, JD, RN, Senior Research Associate, Vanderbilt Institute for Public Policy Studies, 1208 18th Avenue South, Nashville, TN 37212-2099.

4

What is Access and
What Does it Mean for Nursing?

Karen A. Bonuck, M.S.W., M.P.A.
Peter S. Arno, Ph.D.

Montefiore Medical Center/Albert Einstein College of Medicine

Stevens' paper discusses the role of nursing in an inequitable market-driven health care system and offers a conceptualization of access to care. Nurses provide the bulk of primary care and are thus witness to the deleterious effects of limited accessibility to health care. Despite their firsthand knowledge of the health care system's inequities, the profession has largely ignored the social, economic and political conditions that obstruct access to care. If nursing does not transcend its individualistic focus, Stevens cautions, the discipline will be left in a state of theoretical and practical standstill.

 While nurses are in a unique position to gather data for informing public policy on access to health care, this is not often done. In today's world, budget sheets dictate policy, and numbers are political bullets. It is therefore critical for nurses— and all health care practitioners—to systematically document the nature and frequency of barriers to their clients' receipt of health services. Initiatives supported by quantitative data will be more effective in influencing policy than positions based on subjective or anecdotal reports.

Nursing practice and research can illustrate that clinical impacts of delayed treatment ultimately have economic repercussions. As nurses well know, when people are deterred from seeking timely care, existing problems are exacerbated and new ones invariably develop. Delayed care has been associated with longer hospitalizations over a broad spectrum of conditions (Weissman, Stern, Fielding, & Epstein, 1991). Costly use of emergency rooms for primary care among the poor and in areas with few primary care providers is common. A survey of nine low-income communities in New York found the number of primary care visits occurring in emergency rooms was two to four times higher than in other city areas (Community Service Society, 1989). The literature on access to health care has most recently examined how access to specific services affects health outcomes. The incidence of illness, the likelihood of receiving specialized services while hospitalized, and mortality have all been associated with insurance coverage and income (Davis, 1991).

37

To integrate equitable access to health care into nursing's agenda, research efforts such as those indicated above are imperative. Although Stevens lays the theoretical groundwork for further action to ensure equitable access, the broad actions outlined at the end of the article need to be concretized. Nursing education is a critical avenue for reform. It is during the educational process that professionals undergo what the French term 'déformation professionnelle'—literally a deformation of the professional self. Davis (1968), for example, has documented how a recruit's view of the job changes during nurses' professional education. During this socialization, new recruits should be sensitized to systemic issues obstructing patients' achievement of optimal health. The curriculum could be modified to incorporate more information on the sociopolitical context in which practice occurs. Further, practica or projects in which nursing students isolate barriers to health care in their practice and suggest strategies for reform would be useful exercises. Stevens is concerned with the geographical accessibility of services. For example, students may observe elderly patients not attending clinic because the bus schedules are inconvenient for them. Students could gather data on the problem and devise a strategy for attempting to modify either the bus route or clinic hours.

Nursing education must incorporate the realities in which nurses practice and do research. The gap between nursing theory and practice noted by Stevens is evidence that such integration has not yet occurred. Politics play a critical role in shaping this country's response to health care issues. Access, in fact, has been termed a political rather than an operational idea (Aday & Anderson, 1974). The case of AIDS is illustrative. Consider that until 1985 President Reagan had not spoken the word "AIDS" in a formal, public setting (American Foundation for AIDS Research, 1991). Therefore, the first barriers persons with AIDS had to overcome in the epidemic's early days were political and social. Inattention to AIDS, spawned by a lack of national leadership and negative attitudes toward persons initially affected, delayed this country's response to the epidemic. Until AIDS was recognized as a "social problem," funding and programs aimed at providing appropriate services to persons with AIDS were virtually nonexistent.

Political will, in addition to components of equitable health care frequently cited, is an essential first step to meeting peoples' needs. Health insurance and health care's emergence as a social problem has renewed political interest in health care reform. The campaign of Pennsylvania Senator Harris Wofford, a relative political unknown, helped to propel affordable health care to the national agenda when he defeated President Bush's Attorney General Richard Thornburgh in his bid for the Senate seat. Given a political climate where a position on health care reform has become de rigeur among presidential hopefuls, the present is an opportune time for the nursing profession to enter this public policy debate.

The study of access to health care, that is, who receives it, who does not receive it, and why, has been a primary focus of health services researchers. Two theoretical frameworks have dominated the discussion. One, the Health Belief model, places great emphasis on personal characteristics and subjective phenomena affecting health care behavior. The other, the Health Behavior model, in contrast, focuses on barriers to health care posed by economic and sociostructural factors.

The Health Belief model was initially studied in conjunction with preventive health behavior (Rosenstock, 1966). It has since been expanded to include other behaviors such as health care-seeking, sick role and compliance behaviors. Cultural traits (Spector, 1979; Zborowski, 1952; Zola, 1966), class differences (Suchman, 1972), and psychological characteristics (Mechanic, 1974) are considered important determinants in this model. These are the individualistic behaviors which Stevens states nurses must transcend in order to improve access to care. The nursing profession has generally neglected the variables health services researchers and economists have emphasized— financial resources and the accessibility of providers. Individualistic or subjective phenomena obviously play an important role in health care behavior. According to health services researchers, utilization differences attributed to them have, however, been less prominent than differences due to economic and socio-structural variables (Dutton, 1978; Kohler-Reissman, 1974; Kohler-Reissman, 1984; Mechanic, 1989; Wolinsky, 1978).

The Health Behavior model operationalizes access to care in terms of factors predicting the utilization of health services (Aday & Andersen, 1974). These factors include demographic variables related to morbidity, socioeconomic status, insurance, and characteristics of the delivery system, among others. Characteristics of the delivery system, apart from its geographic accessibility to which the author refers, affect access to care. For instance, having a regular source of care has been a strong and consistent predictor of health care utilization. Having a usual source of care, such as a private physician rather than an outpatient clinic, an emergency room, or other hospital-based sources of care, is associated with more frequent utilization (Cornelius, Beauregard, & Cohen, 1991).

Where care is sought affects the treatment received and the "user friendliness" of that source. Care for the poor is concentrated in emergency rooms or hospital outpatient departments rather than private physician offices. These venues tend to be characterized by long waits, short visits, and indifferent or brusque attention. Ease of entry to the health care system also affects its accessibility. Indicators of ease of entry include the transportation mode taken to the source of care, travel time, office waiting time, and waiting time for appointments. There is less ease of entry for minorities, the poor, the uninsured and those persons with a poorer health status in general (Cornelius, Beauregard, & Cohen, 1991).

Stevens amply documents the barriers to health care that inadequate income and insurance pose. While access problems are often income related, interactions between income and other factors also influence access to care. Dutton (1978), for example, found that type of usual source of care, though related to income, has effects independent of it in explaining use of health services by the poor.

Similarly, it has been reported that racial minorities and the poor, with or without appointments, wait longer at private doctors' offices as well as at clinics (Schwartz, 1978). Lower socioeconomic status has also been associated with delays in seeking care, although relatively few patients attributed delays to the cost of care (Weissman, Stern, Fielding, & Epstein, 1991).

According to Stevens, in their theory, practice, and research, nurses should continually be asking "who has access?" Knowing who has access, however, provides an incomplete assessment of the problem. Understanding *why* people do not receive access to health care is as important for guiding corrective actions as knowing *who* does not. Factors or barriers limiting access are the hard data needed for policy and planning. For example, barriers that are amenable to policy control (e.g., coverage of services under Medicaid) can be a practical starting point for implementing measures to improve access to care. On the other hand, prejudices and discrimination toward specific groups (i.e., persons of color, gays and lesbians) which adversely affect the quality of their health care stem from value judgments which are more resistant to change.

Finally, one must also ask if particular services are not routinely received, does this signify a mismatch between supply and demand? Fuchs (1974) refers to these gaps as general access problems because they are experienced by no particular group in society. In this case, asking "what services are unavailable or [what services] do persons generally experience difficulties obtaining," would be more appropriate questions than merely knowing "who has access." Until the explosive growth of the home-care industry in the 1980s, home care was relatively unavailable to most people. Similarly, problems in obtaining AIDS-related drugs were initially experienced by most persons with AIDS because of delays in the search for treatments (Arno & Feiden, 1992).

Access to health care must be understood as a multidimensional issue. The triage rationing referred to by Stevens, an invidious reality for health care providers, is one of many rationing processes. Providers' recognition of a patient's constraints may lead them to balance their need to see a patient frequently with the patient's ability to pay. Institution-specific rationing occurs as high prices of pharmaceuticals lead hospitals to choose between medication alternatives. While many of these drugs offer only negligible improvements over a previously used therapy, in a few instances the newer drugs may save lives or decrease costly hospital stays (Rosenthal, 1991). Rationing by rule may begin on the state level; Oregon has proposed a schema for prioritizing Medicaid services eligible for reimbursement.

The dissatisfaction experienced by nurses who wish to be caregivers but whose jobs frequently dictate that they be gatekeepers is shared by other disciplines. Analogies can be drawn to another field imbued with the ideology of caring, social work. Both are frequently conflicted between the dictates of the constrained organizations they are affiliated with and the welfare of those they serve. This conflict, to which Stevens attributes some attrition from the field, has similarly led to burn-out among social workers. Social policy theorists Cloward and Piven (1975) comment that the emergence of the welfare state (including Medicaid and Medicare) enhanced rather than curbed capitalist health care institutions:

> We had been fundamentally mistaken in our belief that health care institutions, and the professionals attached to them, knew how to help people and urgently wanted to do so. We began to understand that these institutions were shaped by quite different impulses, by the impulses for expansion and profit.

One difference between the two professions is that social work experiences a dialectical tension between individual and systems-oriented change. Nursing, in contrast, has largely remained at the individual level and not experienced this tension.

Playing a role in the attainment of a more equitable health care system is the primary challenge Stevens poses to the nursing profession. Success in attaining this goal will depend partially on the existence of a community spirit in which all parties subscribe to the notion of a social contract. Historically, American social policy has discriminated between the deserving and nondeserving, while individually, persons invariably place themselves among the deserving. We have seen this dichotomization with AIDS, for example, where a number of public figures have attempted to divide persons with AIDS into those who "brought it upon themselves" and "innocent victims." Thus while Stevens states, "most people in the United States believe that everyone is entitled to health care," it is less certain that absolute equity is a principle most Americans currently endorse.

There is, of course, no easy answer. Even in countries with national health care, the presence of queues, private hospitals, and private insurance means that some consumers wait longer for procedures or don't receive them at all. Moreover, it is important not to lose sight of the fact that improving access to health care, while a step in the right direction, is a limited one. It is abundantly clear that in Western European countries, where equitable access is far more a part of the cultural and political landscape than in America, dramatic differentials in health status and life expectancy (by social class) not only remain but have widened in recent years (Balarajan, 1989; Wilkinson, 1992). It is probably a mistake, therefore, for the debate in health care policy reform to focus exclusively on improving access to care. A broader vision is needed—one that includes changes in the environmental and social conditions under which we live—conditions which seem to have a far greater impact on health status than health care itself.

REFERENCES

Aday, L., & Andersen, R. (1974). A framework for studying access to medical care. *Health Services Research, 9,* 208–220.

American Foundation for AIDS Research. (1991). Personal communication.

Arno, P., & Feiden, K. (1992). *Against the odds: The story of AIDS, drug development, politics & profits.* New York: HarperCollins.

Balarajan, R. (1989). Inequalities in health within the health sector. *British Medical Journal, 299,* 822–825.

Cloward, R., & Piven, F. (1975). R. Bailey & M, Brake (Eds.), *Introduction to radical social work* (p. ix). *New York:* Pantheon Press.

Community Service Society. (1989). *Building primary health care in low income communties: Primary health care shortage in nine low income communities.* New York: Author.

Cornelius, L., Beauregard, K., & Cohen, J. (1991). National medical expenditure survey: Usual sources of care and their characteristics. *Research Findings 11.* Agency for Health Care Policy and Research. Rockville, MD: Public Health Service.

Davis, F. (1968). Professional socialization as subjective experience: The process of doctrinal conversion among nursing students. In Becker, H., et al., *Institutions and the person* (pp. 235–251). Chicago: Aldine.

Davis, K. (1991). Inequality and access to health care. *The Milbank Quarterly, 69,* 253–273.

Dutton, D. (1978). Explaining the low use of health services by the poor: Costs, attitudes, or delivery systems. *American Sociological Review, 43,* 348–368.

Fuchs, V. (1974). *Who shall live? Health, economics and social choice.* New York: Basic Books.

Kohler-Reissman, C. (1974). The use of health services by the poor. *Social Policy, May/June,* 41–49.

Kohler-Reissman, C. (1984). The use of health services by the poor: Are there any promising models. *Social Policy, Spring,* 30–40.

Mechanic, D. (1974). Social psychologic factors affecting the presentation of bodily complaints. In *Politics, medicine, and social science.* New York: John Wiley & Sons.

Mechanic, D. (1989). Correlates of physician utilization: Why do major multivariate studies of physician utilization find trivial psychosocial and organizational effects. In *Painful choices: Research and essays on health care* (pp. 135–150). New Brunswick, NJ: Transaction Publishers.

Rosenstock, I. (1966). Why people use health services. *Milbank Memorial Quarterly Fund, 44,* 94–127.

Rosenthal, E. (1991, December 18). As costs of new drugs rise, hospitals stick by old ones. *New York Times,* p. A-1.

Schwartz, B. (1978). The social ecology of time barriers. *Social Forces, 56,* 1203–1220.

Spector, R. (1979). Ethnicity and health: A study of health care beliefs and practices. *Urban and Social Change Review, 12,* 34–37.

Suchman, E. (1972). Social patterns of illness and medical care. In E. G. Jaco (Ed.), *Patients, physicians and illness* (pp. 262–279). New York: The Free Press.

Weissman, J., Stern, R., Fielding, S., & Epstein, A. (1991). Delayed access to health care: Risk factors, reasons, and consequences. *Annals of Internal Medicine, 114,* 325–331.

Wilkinson, R. (1992). Education and debate: Income distribution and life expectancy. *British Medical Journal, 304,* 165–168.

Wolinsky, F. (1978). Assessing the effects of predisposing, enabling and illness-morbidity characteristics on health service utilization. *Journal of Health and Social Behavior, 19,* 384–396.

Zborowski, M. (1952). Cultural components in response to pain. *Journal of Social Issues, 8,* 16–30.

Zola, I. (1966). Culture and symptoms—An analysis of patients' presenting complaints. *American Sociological Review, 31,* 615–630.

Offprints. Requests for offprints should be sent to Karen A. Bonuck, M.S.W., M.P.A., Department of Epidemiology and Social Medicine, Montefiore Medical Center, Albert Einstein College of Medicine, 111 East 210th Street, Bronx, NY 10467-2490.

5

Who Will Pay?
The Economic Realities of
Health Care Reform

Carolyne K. Davis, Ph.D., R.N., F.A.A.N.[1]

Ernst & Young

Stevens' paper contributes to an increased awareness of nurses' responsibilities toward access to care. The paper is well documented to enhance the premise that everyone in the United States is entitled to health care. While the author identifies several strategies that can and must be carried out in order to influence change, the paper lacks clarity in the more practical aspects of economic realities such as who will pay for these increased services.

In placing pressure on groups such as health care institutions, insurance companies, and government to make changes, we fail to recognize that the general public still has not indicated a willingness to pay for universal access to health care. While most polls show interest in expanding health care coverage to include the uninsured and underinsured, less than a majority of individuals have indicated a willingness to pay more than $100 to expand coverage to these groups (Hart/ Teeter Poll, 1991). It seems apparent that an educational campaign will thus be necessary to convince the general public of the need for more comprehensive state and national health care programs for which each citizen will have to pay, even if indirectly through taxes.

One area that should be identified for research and practice is the economics of cost/benefit analysis. As nurses, we are responsible for assuring that each dollar spent is spent wisely and that supplies and equipment are not wasted. Inefficiencies in care must be identified not only to improve the quality of care but to reduce the cost. Economic necessity dictates that even if we were to achieve a consensus about universal access to health care, we would need to couple this with economical nursing practice. Too few nurses are willing to be a part of this solution by utilizing research and practice to identify outcomes of care linked to best practice. Yet these activities must be a part of the future of nursing, if we are to achieve the necessary savings to provide for expanded coverage.

---

[1] F.A.A.N. until 1985.

Insurance companies are attempting to work with state insurance commissions as well as the federal government to secure relief so that they can adequately offer insurance options to small group employers. Current regulatory controls over the insurance industry have prevented the latter from being able to adequately respond to consumer needs. By understanding these issues, nurses can join with consumer groups and insurance organizations in lobbying to change the excessive regulatory environment.

Employers everywhere are experiencing significant increases in their health care benefits programs. While they are spending many more dollars than before as a percent of total payroll, they are also asking employees to share the burden by assuming increased co-payments and deductibles, as well as increased premiums. This awareness of the cost of health care has created the current climate of concern regarding not only access to care, but also the spiraling cost of health care delivery.

A careful study of other countries' systems of universal health care indicates that countries with universal health care are also struggling with issues such as cost and access. For example, the growth in actual per capita spending between 1980–1987 shows that Canada, with a 9.9% compound annual growth rate, is actually ahead of the United States with its 9.4% rate, while the United Kingdom trails slightly with 9.3% (Scheiber & Poullier, 1989). Long waiting times or queuing for elective surgery has long been recognized as a component of the United Kingdom universal health coverage system, but has only recently been reported in the Canadian system (Detsky, 1990; Litton, 1990; Walker, 1991).

"Invisible rationing" is not a product of the U.S. health care system alone, but rather occurs in some fashion in almost every system—even Canada and the United Kingdom with their universal health care (Scheiber & Poullier, 1989). The basic fact is that new technology is developing faster than any society appears to be willing and able to pay for it. A review of European countries indicates an attempt to control outlays for health care. Rationing, price controls, and increased co-payments and deductibles or increased premiums are becoming a way of life in most developed nations today.

One fact is clear—all other countries have better access to primary care delivery than we have in the United States. Central to any type of health care system reform for us should be the importance of developing better primary care delivery. This is an area where nursing needs to be involved, not only in the development of policy but also in the provision of primary care services.

The utopian premise that everyone must get all the health care that he/she needs and wants will be difficult to sell to a society that is not yet convinced that we in the health care sector have done all that we can to assure the maximum cost-effective use of current resources. Nursing must indeed be concerned with equitable access to high-quality, nondiscriminatory health care. Stevens identifies several nursing responsibilities that will enhance the ability of nursing to be a part of the policy arena that will develop this new system. Many alternative plans will be developed and debated during the next several years. Nursing must be a significant voice in these debates.

REFERENCES

Blue Cross of California. (1990). *Health care in the 90's: A global view of delivery and financing.*

Detsky, A. (1990). Canada's system of health insurance. In *Health care in the 90's: A global view of delivery and financing* (p. 30). Blue Cross of California.

Linton, A. L. (1990). Canadian health care: A physician's perspective. In *Health care in the 90's: A global view of delivery and financing.* Blue Cross of California.

Hart/Teeter Poll (#4023). (1991, June). *NBC/Wall Street Journal.*

Scheiber, G. J., & Poullier, J. P. (1989, Fall). International health care expenditure trends: 1987. *Health Affairs,* p. 174.

Scheiber, G. J., & Poullier, J. P. (1989). Our view of internal comparisons of health care expenditure. In *International comparisons of health care financing and delivery—health care financing review. 1989 Annual supplement.* Baltimore, MD: Health Care Financing Administration, U.S. Department of Health and Human Services.

Walder, M. (1991, October 16). Personal communication. The Fraser Institute, Vancouver, British Columbia.

Offprints. Requests for offprints should be directed to Dr. Carolyne Davis, c/o Ernst & Young, 1200 19th Street, N.W., Suite 400, Washington, DC 20036.

6

Nursing's Proposal
for Health Care Reform

Lucille A. Joel, Ed.D., R.N., F.A.A.N.

Rutgers, The State University of New Jersey

Equitable access to health care is a fundamental belief of nursing. Reform of America's health care system to provide access to essential services will require restructuring the delivery arrangement for services. The triad of access, quality, and cost is among the fundamental reforms that America's nurses envision.

Heroics and sophisticated technology save lives. But by failing to provide universal access to essential primary health care, preventable illnesses flourish and chronic diseases become a way of life.

Unequal access cannot be reconciled with desired emphasis on prevention and early intervention. Nurses recognize that reforms must be viewed within a larger social, economic and political context. Poverty, exposure to illicit drugs, inadequate nutrition, and poor education individually and collectively contribute to poor health. Unacceptable infant mortality rates, increasing teen suicide rates, chronic substance abuse problems, and the spread of preventable diseases, including measles, tuberculosis and HIV, fuel the skyrocketing costs of health care.

In 1990, the national health bill was 12.4% of the Gross National Product. Analysts expect that amount to rise 12% to 15% a year. At that rate, it would reach nearly $1.8 trillion in 1995 and nearly $2.7 trillion by the year 2000 (Bowsher, 1991). In 1989, health care benefits cost companies $2,700 per employee. In 1990 this figure exceeded $3,000 (Health Insurance Association of America, 1990). There are 34 million people uninsured and of this number 20 million are employees and dependents who work for small businesses (Meyer, Sullivan, & Silow-Carroll, 1991).

As these problems push health care and insurance costs higher, more organized groups are getting involved in the health care reform movement. Each group has its own agenda, although recently business has joined providers, consumers, insurance companies, and legislators as participants in the debate over resolving the problems that plague America's health care system (Miller, 1991). Among its other positions, business has voiced concern about the access and quality of services, most notably as they affect pregnant women and their children—

America's future workers and employees (National Leadership Coalition for Health Care Reform, 1991).

Nursing is in a position to define the factors that create the system's problems and to identify the most efficacious resolutions to those problems. The result of the profession's unique insight and expertise is *Nursing's Agenda for Health Care Reform* (American Nurses Association, 1991), a plan that is realistic, practical and based on first-hand understanding of what needs to be done. The Agenda presents a comprehensive health policy plan that addresses access, quality of care, financing, and implementation. It is a bold new vision for reform—one that keeps what works best in our current system but casts aside institutions and policies that fail to meet present and future needs. It calls for no new dollars, but for the reallocation of existing dollars.

Nursing's agenda calls for universal access to a federally defined package of basic health benefits. Access would be guaranteed through a new delivery structure that would emphasize managed care and care delivered in convenient, familiar, community-based sites such as schools and the workplace. Consumers would be encouraged to take more responsibility for their own health, with health care providers educating them about healthful behaviors. At the same time, consumers would have access to a full range of qualified health care professionals to allow for necessary, therapeutically effective care at an affordable price.

By mandating a core of health care services that are accessible to all residents, nursing's agenda would reduce the incidence of preventable illnesses that drain the financial coffers to serve a few while basic care is being denied to many. Savings would accrue by avoiding the expenses associated with treating conditions that could have been prevented. It is known that every $1 spent in immunizations can save $3 in treating communicable childhood illnesses.

Nursing's plan would control costs of health care through re-allocating dollars saved from administrative and bureaucratic costs, defensive and unnecessary medical practices, and fragmented services. Other steps to increase access and reduce the costs of health care include the utilization of a full range of qualified providers, controlled growth of the health care system through planning and prudent resource allocation, and increased use of case management that promotes consumers' active participation in their care. A public plan would be accessible to all citizens with incomes below 200% of the poverty line, and affordable to small business and individuals who would choose to subscribe. This plan would mandate managed care.

All individuals offered private plans as employment benefits would be encouraged to use managed systems. Public and private funding for long-term care services would prevent personal impoverishment resulting from serious, chronic or degenerative illness. Insurance reforms would assure improved access to coverage, including affordable premiums and reinsurance pools for catastrophic situations.

If all of these reforms are adopted the collective health will improve and a savings will result. Fully implemented, *Nursing's* plan for reform would restructure America's health delivery system to emphasize the importance of health, consumer empowerment, and sensitivity to local need.

REFERENCES

American Nurses Association. (1991). *Nursing's agenda for health care reform.* Kansas City, MO: Author.

Bowsher, C. A. (1991). *U.S. health care spending: Trends, contributing factors and proposals for reform.* Statement before the Committee on Ways and Means, House of Representatives. Washington, D.C.

Health Insurance Association of America (1990). *Source book of health insurance data.* Washington, DC: Author.

Meyer, J., Sullivan, S., & Silow-Carroll, S. (March 1991). *Private sector initiatives: Controlling health care costs.* Washington, DC: Health Care Leadership Council.

Miller, R. S. (1991). *Reform of the health care system. Statement of the Chrysler Corporation before the Senate Committee on Finance, Subcommittee on Health for Families and the Uninsured.* Washington, DC.

The National Leadership Coalition for Health Care (1991). *Excellent health care for all Americans at a reasonable cost: A proposal for three-dimensional health care reform.* Washington, DC: Author.

Offprints. Requests for offprints should be sent to Lucille A. Joel, Ed.D., R.N., F.A.A.N., 594 Blauvelt Drive, Oradell, NJ 07649.

7

A Political Perspective
on Health Care Access

Joel S. Levine, M.D.

University of Colorado Health Sciences Center, Denver

The principal focus of this response will be to place this paper into the broad political economic context in which change will ultimately be fashioned. In the absence of our having a system of government that can mandate change in our health care delivery 'system,' such as occurred in Cuba or China, we must deal with the complexities and realities of our representative, nonparliamentary form of government, whose powers were purposely separated to reduce the chance of radical change. This is the imperfect court in which such issues are adjudicated in the United States. Any attempt to change our health care delivery system must take into account several realities: (a) politicians are uncertain about what their constituents are saying, (b) powerful special interest groups provide clear messages to Congress and the President, and (c) real change will require an acceptance of the fiscal realities of late-twentieth century America and a willingness to compromise.

On a superficial level what 'we' tell our politicians seems pretty clear, with 85% of those polled expressing such deep dissatisfaction with our current system of health care delivery that they want some type of extensive change (Taylor & Reinhardt, 1991). Once we get away from the fact that 'we' are unhappy about the current state of affairs, however, the message becomes extremely fuzzy. Most of us believe that the government should assure access to health care for the sick, while also feeling that the government is incapable of managing anything in an efficient manner. We believe that health care costs are too much, while feeling at the same time that not enough resources are spent on high-technology services or care for the terminally ill. We want to expand access to the uninsured, but some of us who are healthy and earn an income are unwilling to be taxed for this expansion. Those polled prefer the concept of a Canadian system. Would voters in this country be willing to have a 46% upper-tax bracket and a 7% value-added tax (essentially a federal sales tax), however, as occurs in Canada? In view of these inconsistencies it is no surprise that politicians have been squeamish about trying to put out the health care delivery fire. They're afraid that either they will put out the wrong fire or be given gasoline by some well-meaning health services researcher. The memory of Medicare Catastrophic Insurance will be long and deep.

In contrast to the fuzzy messages of their constituents, the voices of advocacy groups and lobbyists are crystal clear. Unfortunately, they are also commonly irreconcilable. The voices for 'fine-tuning' of the current system have come from those who benefit most from the status quo: the providers (doctors, hospitals, for-profit health care systems), small businesses that do not provide insurance, and the insurers. Included within these groups is much of the $60-100 billion in 'administrative waste' that is put forward as the source of funds for insuring the uninsured with the conversion to a single-payer (tax-based, government-run) system (GAO Report, 1991). It needs to be recognized that this 'waste' is largely composed of 3-to-5 million people working for a living as insurance agents, claims adjusters, quality assurance reviewers, utilization managers, collection agencies, etc. These individuals are politically savvy and block-vote on special interests. Small businesses getting a free ride by not providing insurance are very effective lobbyists. In addition, these groups control (directly and indirectly) much of the wealth and resources of this country that are not currently owned by the Japanese and Europeans. Against these juggernauts are arrayed a host of small advocacy or special interest groups pushing for a major change in our system. Despite agreeing on the problems, each of these groups has decided that its way is the 'best' way to change the system. The inability of these groups to compromise and develop a consensus has, therefore, tended toward each canceling the other out from a political standpoint. The only reason that the President has been able to remain aloof from this issue is that too many advocacy groups have preferred the status quo as opposed to considering the value of other proposals being offered.

Despite the election year political rhetoric, change of the current delivery system to improve equity and access will be difficult to accomplish in this last decade of the millennium because of the constraints on resource allocation that are now being confronted. The federal government has become increasingly ineffective in the face of more than a $3 trillion deficit whose interest payments cost more than the combined expenditures on Medicare and Medicaid. State governments, unable or unwilling to deficit finance, are being slowly driven into bankruptcy by Medicaid mandates. Worse, some are deciding that these mandates will be paid for by reducing the support for education and other social services that are part of the flexible portion of their budget. This is all occurring at a time when many believe that the deplorable public health statistics (infant mortality, etc.) detailed by Stevens will be improved more by channeling resources into housing, education, and job training rather than into health care delivery. At this time, throwing more money into the health care pot is not an acceptable political alternative.

With an expanding portion of our national wealth going to the health care sector, cost control, not access, is dictating the political agenda. The incremental approaches of the past three decades have failed to keep the overall pace of health lation at or below that of other goods and services. One might question whether the blame for this relative increase in costs lies completely within the health care sector, or is some portion of this discrepancy due to the lack of productivity in the rest of our society? At a time when most of America seems satisfied to utilize their children's inheritance instead of prioritizing their current needs, when potential costs of health care services have no upper limit, and when Americans' expectations of individual access to high technology services seem infinite, one wonders whether cost controls will ever be palatable and politically achievable (Russell, 1989).

Where does this leave individuals, such as Stevens, who feel deeply about the inequities of our current non-system of health care delivery? Stevens has made a good first step in confronting her own profession with the impact of inequitable access on health care outcomes. There is a growing interest in getting health care professionals to examine their own values, and compare them to the actuality of their practice. Stevens challenges the nursing profession to consider the potential conflicts between caregiving and gatekeeping, and between social responsibility and the profit motive. All health care providers would do well to examine the conduct of their professional lives, and the emphasis they have given to caring for patients as opposed to earning a living.

Recognizing that change will be played out in a political arena, an advocate for reform must tie proposals to improve equity to clearly defined ways to control costs, and be willing to be flexible about the 'right' way to achieve these goals. Despite our country's inability in the past to resolve this issue, it shouldn't be that difficult a problem if we look at the rest of the world. Stevens appears particularly intrigued by the Canadian system, the second costliest system per capita in the world. In fact, every other industrialized nation in the world has found a way to do a better job of providing equitable access at lower cost than has the United States. The fascinating thing is that each country has been successful despite apparent differences in delivery structure. A lesson that any advocate can take away is that equity and cost control do not require a single-payer system, a national health service, socialism, or capitation. By the same token, to date, America's competitive, free-market model has failed to provide either universal access or cost control. Are there some general lessons we can learn from the industrialized nations of Europe and Asia? I believe so.

1. Cost control requires universal access.
   This is a simple concept, but one that continues to elude the policy makers. Even the strongest proponents of a competitive, market-driven model have accepted the concept that some level of equitable access is a *necessary* component of any health care system (Enthoven & Kronick, 1989).
2. An equitable system does not require a sole payer, *but* when the system allows multiple insurers they must be willing to insure each citizen with a community rating. The concept of denying health insurance to the ill is perverse.
3. All citizens (old-young, rich-poor, healthy-sick) get the same benefits within the system, with the rich paying more than the poor through the use

of tax-transfers. It is interesting that the current 'system' in the United States provides most of the governmental support for health insurance to the non-poor.

4. Every citizen accepts the responsibility for contributing to, and being, insured. The government accepts the responsibility for the insurance of the poor. This cannot be an optional or individual decision; if it is, the community rating system fails.

5. Medical benefits are not open-ended, and many countries have a greater emphasis on prevention than does America. Most nations allow people to buy insurance for the services that the system does not reimburse.

6. Most countries also put a cap on total expenditures through the use of arbitration with the major providers (hospitals, physicians) and the creation of global budgets.

It is important to note before summarizing my thoughts that nurses with whom I work are not "overlooking glaring social, economic, and political conditions that are detrimental to the population's health." I see them working on the front lines of community and migrant health centers, rural health clinics, and public health services. They are integral parts of the new wave of excellent health services research that has identified the problems that underline Stevens' paper. They are central to the patient and professional advocacy groups that provide some balance to the laws and regulations under which our current system functions. Some have major leadership roles among the staffs of the major health committees in Congress. Indeed, nurses are examining the social, behavioral, and economic forces that modify the presentation, course, and treatment of patients. More of the same is needed.

In summary, then, change in our health care delivery system is inevitable. The ultimate structure of that system is highly conjectural at this time, but hopefully it will take into account some of the unique cultural values of the American people. There are more pressures for change being generated because of the concerns about cost than because of the restriction of access. Therefore, it is imperative that all health care professionals, acting as their patients' advocates, begin to take part in the political process that will create the change.

REFERENCES

Enthoven, A., & Kronick, R., (1989). A consumer choice health plan for the 1990s. New *England Journal of Mediine, 320,* 29–37.

General Accounting Office. (1991). *Canadian health insurance, Lessons for the United States.* Report ERD-91-90. Washington, DC: Author.

Russell, L. B. (1989). Some of the tough decisions required by a national health plan. *Science, 246,* 892–896.

Taylor, H., & Reinhardt, U. E. (1991). Does the system fit? *HMQ, Third Quarter,* 2–10.

Offprints. Requests for offprints should be sent to Joel S. Levine, M.D., Division of Gastroenterology, University of Colorado Health Sciences Center, Box B-158, 4200 E. 9th Avenue, Denver, CO 80262.

8

Qui Bono?
Nursing Education in the
Context of Nursing's Agenda
for Health Care Reform

Patricia Moccia, Ph.D., R.N., F.A.A.N.

National League for Nursing

The nursing community's proactive position on how, where and by whom health care should be delivered will ultimately depend for its success on similar changes in the educational sector. Nursing's proposal for a consumer-driven, community-based system of primary health care providers has called into question long-held beliefs about how, where, and by whom nurses should be educated. In addition to the structural changes proposed in the prevailing delivery system, *Nursing's Agenda for Health Care Reform* calls upon providers—in both community and institutional settings—to radically redefine their clinical practice, loyalties, political allies and power nexus. No less will be expected of nursing education and nurse educators.

The nature of the demand for nurses will change significantly from what has been the case until now as *Nursing's Agenda for Health Care Reform* is successfully advanced at the national and local levels. The *Agenda* proposes changes in structures, practice patterns, financing and the relationships among professionals and between professionals and patients. These changes include an increased emphasis on promotion and prevention services and decreased dependence on technology and medical interventions. The medical monopoly that characterizes the status quo will be disassembled as private and public financing provides direct reimbursement for a range of alternative providers, including nurses; services will be more accessible, delivered in such settings as schools and worksites, community clinics and nursing centers.

If we are to meet this new kind of demand, the supply of nurses will need to differ from the current profile in both numbers and kind. Nurse educators are, therefore, about to undertake the task of designing and/or modifying programs and curricula in order to assure that we can deliver on the promises made within the reforms proposed. At this moment, the questions for nurse educators include where and how to begin.

Before the reform movement in either health care delivery or nursing education is further advanced, however, additional analysis is needed as to both systems' social construction (i.e, how, and by whom, they are developed) and social function (i.e., what purposes they serve in society.) This paper argues that: (a) Stevens' question exposes the social construction of health care but not its social function; (b) *Nursing's Agenda for Health Care Reform* implicitly questions the social function but not the social construction of the delivery System; and (c) while both the social construction and social function of nursing education have been questioned by the "Curriculum Revolution," considerable theoretical work remains to be done relative to higher education in general.

WHICH QUESTIONS EXPOSE WHICH RELATIONSHIPS?

Health care and education are but two of society's mediating systems. Mediating systems are those through which society's values and a culture's mores are transmitted, reproduced and extended. They include both discrete entities such as the legal and penal systems, and the more amorphous ones such as the arts.

In the view of most (but admittedly not all) social analysts, such systems play several roles in addition to their specific functions of, in this case, delivering health care services and preparing individuals for particular professional responsibilities. Within such an understanding, mediating systems are socially constructed to reflect, reinforce, reproduce and extend a society's prevailing ideology. In addition, precisely because they are social constructs, such systems also reflect, reproduce and extend the relationships among any society's constituent parts.

In posing the question: "Who Gets Care," Stevens begins her analysis from an especially illuminating position that advances the socio-political understanding necessary for health care reform to take place. By identifying those denied access—the poor and working class, women and children, individuals from traditionally underrepresented racial and ethnic communities, gays and lesbians—Stevens not only identifies the social inequities of health care, she exposes similar imbalances in society as a whole. Stevens' arguments establish a sound basis for developing nursing research within broad socio-political frameworks; and, so too, for nursing education. Her arguments also allow a broader approach for intervention in the interest of reform than has usually been the case in the nursing community despite the significant work done on our history by authors such as Dock, Wald and Ashley, and work done more recently.

Stevens's arguments, however, rest on two inter-related assumptions which, if questioned, hold even greater potential for the change she argues is needed to achieve the social equality she argues is desired. Arguments for increased access assume that the current health care system is appropriately constructed to meet the health care needs of society, and that increased access to the system would be of benefit to those currently denied. While revealing the social construction of the health care system, such arguments lead us toward solutions that do little to uncover its social function. They are reformist at heart and ignore, whether by design or default, questions of ideology which, when posed, argue for the more fundamental change necessary to assure a healthier society.

THE HEALTH CARE DELIVERY SYSTEM: QUI BONO?

Questions of social function might be posed in several ways in order to uncover the particular ideology being served. For example, while never explicitly calling the dominant ideology into question, *Nursing's Agenda* implies an alternative view of the world through its focus on alternative providers and a consumer-driven system. In so doing, it challenges the status quo.

Others have questioned the health care system with the classic "Qui bono?" "To Whose Good?" In a classic and comprehensive treatise, *The Social Transformation of American Medicine*, Paul Starr (1982) argues that the health care system is structured for the "sole" benefit of (a) organized medicine, and (b) a vast medical-industrial conglomerate of profitable business built on the authority of medicine for the purpose of reinforcing and reproducing medicine's dominance. In her classic, *Hospitals, Paternalism and the Role of the Nurse*, Ashley (1976) questioned the relationships that were the context of nurses' experiences within hospitals and uncovered a structural relationship within the hospital system of paternalism, dependency and, in too many cases, abusive patterns. She argued that a patriarchal ideology was thus served.

Both questions, "Who Has Access?" and "Qui Bono?" are posed with the assumption that the status quo is in need of change and with the intent of identifying the direction or nature of the change needed. The significance of the differences exposed when one begins with Stevens' question of "Who Has Access?" compared to the question "Qui bono?" lies in the different possibilities for action that would logically follow. Stevens' question directs us toward proposals designed to increase the number of individuals who have access, and the number and range of services to which access is to be had. Starr (1982) and Ashley are among those whose questions would lead us to change the nature of the services offered. It is the latter question and its implications that parallel most closely the potential impact of *Nursing's Agenda for Health Care Reform*.

NURSING AND HIGHER EDUCATION: QUI BONO?

Few would debate that, as a mediating system, higher education is both socially constructed and serves a social function. The "Who Has Access" question has been posed for higher education but not yet for nursing education. For example, there are widely recognized analyses that community colleges, rather than serving as an avenue of social mobility, serve to "cool out" individual aspirations and aggregate demands for access. There is also a growing recognition that, as currently structured, higher education serves an ideology of a different era and is, therefore, in need of significant structural change.

Considerable attention has been paid to reforming pedagogy and the experiences of nursing education via a "curriculum revolution" or the transformation of programs developed within the traditionalist Tylerian model [Allen (1990), Bevis & Murray (1990), deTornyay (1990), Diekelmann (1990), Tanner (1990), Waters (1990)]. Yet to be thoroughly questioned, in a way similar to Ashley's analysis, are the structural relationships which support the "unreal loyalties" between educators and systems of higher education. Before planning for any reform in nursing education to parallel *Nursing's Agenda*, similar questions of the dominant ideology need to be posed, as in the delivery sector, to identify possible actions to be taken.

Clearly, as the *Agenda* is advanced, nursing education will need to be changed. But toward what end and via which avenues? These questions depend on the fundamental "Qui bono" nursing education? Or in Virginia Woolf's words: "Where is it leading us, the procession of educated men?" (Woolf, 1938).

SUMMARY

Stevens' question "Who Gets Care?" is in the tradition of those arguing for increased access and a more equitable distribution of society's benefits. As such, it provides a framework for nursing scholarship concerned with social as contrasted with individual interventions. *Nursing's Agenda for Health Care Reform* advances the argument still further by questioning the ideology reinforced by the current system, and offering an alternative system, alternative services and agents. In so doing, the proposed agenda questions the dominant ideology and is, therefore, more accurately a radical departure from the status quo than a reform. While there are some implicit assumptions of both reform and radical change embedded within the work of those addressing a "curriculum revolution," the discussion would benefit from explicit expositions of both the social construction and social function of higher education.

REFERENCES

Allen, D. (1990). The curriculum revolution: Radical re-visioning of nursing education. *Journal of Nursing Education, 29*(7), 312–317.

Ashley, J. (1976). *Hospitals, paternalism and the role of the nurse.* New York: Teachers College Press.

Bovis, E., & Murray, J. (1990). The essence of the curriculum revolution: Emancipatory teaching. *Journal of Nursing Education, 29*(7), 326–331.

deTornyay, R. (1990). The curriculum revolution. *Journal of Nursing Education, 29*(7), 292–294.

Diskelmann, N. (1990). Nursing education: Caring, dialogue, and practice. *Journal of Nursing Education, 29*(7), 300–306.

Starr, P. (1982). *Social transformation of American medicine.* New York: Basic Books.

Tanner, C. (1990). Reflections on the curriculum revolution. *Journal of Nursing Education, 29*(7), 295–299.

Waters, V. (1990). Associate degree nursing and curriculum revolution. *Journal of Nursing Education, 29*(7), 322–325.

Woolf, V. (1938). *Three guineas.* New York: Harcourt, Brace, Jovanovich.

Offprints. Requests for offprints should be sent to Patricia Moccia, Ph.D., R.N., F.A.A.N., National League for Nursing, 350 Hudson Street, New York, NY 10014.

9

Equality vs. Individuality: American Values in Conflict

James Muyskens, Ph.D.

University of Kansas

THE TRAGEDY OF NO ACCESS IN A LAND OF PLENTY

Imagine yourself an intergalactic traveler exploring how the inhabitants of various settlements address their health care needs. You are about to land on planet earth, and your first stop will be New York City. Your guide reminds you that the country you are about to enter has great wealth and has had astonishing success in the development of medical treatment modalities. Vast sums have been spent to develop techniques to rescue accident victims, patients with organ failure, and sufferers of infectious diseases. Many people who in the recent past would have died can now be saved through the "miracle" of high-tech medicine.

Your tour takes you to the major medical centers of metropolitan New York and the neighborhoods in which these centers are located. You discover, however, that large numbers of the people living en route have no access to the care provided in these centers. Your first hypothesis is that the society you are visiting must have a caste system and an ideology to support it. You quickly learn, however, that this society proclaims itself to be egalitarian, and takes pride in being a land of opportunity for all. In the harbor, on the Statue of Liberty, you read the inscription:

> *Give me your tired, your poor,*
> *Your huddled masses yearning to breathe free,*
> *The wretched refuse of your teeming shore.*
> *Send these, the homeless, tempest-tost to me,*
> *I lift my lamp beside the golden door!*

You are told that one of this country's most cherished myths is that, no matter how humble in birth, anyone born in this country can rise to the presidency.

You soon learn that it is a matter of great concern that so many citizens' lives are not enriched by the presence of the best medical services on the planet. National and state legislators are being pressed to solve the problem. Politicians are making campaign promises and bold statements. The topic is on everyone's lips.

As in all the other societies you have studied, you realize that ideology plays a crucial role. In this case, contrary to your first impressions that you had encountered a society with a class-based ideology, you now see that the opposite is true. The deep-seated American commitments to equality and individual advancement are driving forces.

Paradoxically, the egalitarian ideology, combined with uniquely American frontier values, appears to work against meaningful change. This immigrant and frontier society that has eschewed limits cannot reconcile itself to the fact that vast numbers of its citizens are living under oppressive limits. Other societies, perhaps less idealistic and less wealthy, are better able to face the fact that there are limits. They consciously and deliberately develop health care delivery systems that ration care.

Rationing sounds evil, if not "un-American," to American ears. As more and more becomes possible through advances in technology, the limits, however, to what we can afford are becoming tighter. It becomes more and more difficult to deny that some things are simply beyond our reach. Thus, the rationing that does take place occurs as far from view as possible.

Rationing begins *outside* the clinic or medical center door with something so basic as the inability to pay. Typically, our self-respect predisposes us to say as little as possible to others about our ability to pay for what is needed and wanted. When the situation is not desperate, we would sooner forgo something than be put into a position of having to "admit to the world" that we lack the resources. Thus, only a small percentage of the cases of denial of care due to inability to pay is visible beyond a very small circle of acquaintances. The invisible rationing occurs *inside* as well. Limitations of staff, space, and resources in many ways determine who will be served and who will not be served.

The result is that some citizens are served very well. The rationing on both the outside and the inside has no adverse effect upon them. Other citizens are served poorly and must live with the anxiety that comes from knowing that any turn of fate can result in financial ruin and loss of health. In increasing numbers, poorly served citizens wait powerlessly as a treatable problem turns into a life-threatening condition before it is finally possible to get grudging attention in an overcrowded, understaffed public hospital.

Your report, written as you embark for another destination, will state that, despite notable success and noble intentions, the U.S. health care delivery system is dehumanizing, exploitive, and cost-ineffective. You also issue a warning. You point out that, despite long-standing commitments to the contrary, the U.S. is fast becoming tolerant of poverty, discrimination, and the presence of a permanent underclass. You conclude by asking rhetorically whether this is the kind of society Americans want.

PROVIDING ACCESS TO A DECENT MINIMUM OF HEALTH CARE

Clearly, the society we are becoming, due, in part, to the crisis in health care, is not what we want or what our founders had in mind. We can and we must do better. Stevens has done an admirable job outlining the problem of access and offering an account of equitable access. She goes on to indicate how nurses can play a significant role in achieving the goal. This response challenges her view that we must establish a system that can deliver equitable access. Instead, it settles for a more modest goal of providing a decent minimum of health care to all. Full support is given to her view that nurses can and should be active in this reform movement. The notion of collective responsibility is introduced as a way of supplementing her discussion.

In the imaginary scene in the beginning, we were able to stand back from our situation and view it from afar. We saw the centrality of the fundamental commitment to equality. Stevens builds her case for access on this foundation. She wants nothing less than the same for everyone. As she sees it, any differences that favor one over another are insidious.

To argue against such a position is, in a sense, to argue against America, motherhood, and apple pie. Yet, it is important to do so. For, as hinted above, paradoxically, an absolute commitment to equality appears to be getting in the way of a realistic approach to the gross inequalities that plague us.

The standards for access to health care espoused by Stevens set a much higher standard for health care than we set for other basic goods, for example, education, police and fire protection, and environmental safety. The equitable access that she demands includes: (a) relative costs of health care are experienced equally across all groups; (b) health care availability is based on the health needs and geographic distribution of the population rather than on the distribution of wealth; and (c) health care encounters are of equal quality and comprehensiveness across all groups. While valuable as an ideal toward which to strive, it is immobilizing if advanced as a standard that must be realized here and now. The unbridgable gap between what is demanded and what is possible results in denial of the very real conditions of scarcity that constrain us.

The notion that must be added to Stevens' discussion is that of a "decent minimum" of health care services. This is in contrast either to equity or equality of health care services. The contrast can perhaps best be illustrated by looking at education. We believe that it is a right of every child to go to school and acquire an education. Certain standards and minimums must be satisfied or we have failed the student. What is not required, however, is that whatever is possible for some must be made available to all; nor does this entitlement extend beyond a certain basic level (high school graduation).

While the analogy is apt, it must be admitted that it is much easier to delineate what we mean by providing a basic education than it is to specify what does and does not constitute a basic level of health care. In recent years, the struggle for such a definition has been most dramatic in the State of Oregon. The painful steps taken by the citizens of Oregon will soon be taken by others as well. None of us will be able to escape the fact that not all the good that can be done is affordable. To go beyond these general remarks concerning medical economics in this essay, however, would take us too far afield.

In a frontier country such as ours we are not willing to settle for anything less than the optimal without a fight. While not yet recognized by all, that fight is now over, and the time has come to recognize the limits. What we must not give up, however, even if we must give up our utopian dreams, is our commitment to fairness and respect for the value of each individual. Contrary to what may seem to be the case, the lesser alternative advanced in this response is consistent with our sense of fair play and justice.

When each and every member of a group gets what he or she needs, while some get more than they need, no one has thereby been wronged. Suppose, for example, that the unequal distribution provides an incentive to those who get extra, and that this surplus ends up benefiting the whole. Consider the following thought experiment: What "world" would be preferable? World One in which all 50 inhabitants have equal shares (two each) for a grand total of 100 units, or World Two in which no one has less than two shares, but several members have two and a half or three for a collective total of 110 units. If equality is paramount, World One must be selected. Yet most of us would favor World Two because we would recognize that, unless the less fortunate suffer from envy, no one is worse off in World Two than in World One, while some are better off.

How does this apply to our current situation? Despite an egalitarian ideology, our country has vast differences in individual wealth. If we must bring the fortunate few down to the level of the masses, we will join a political fight with very long odds. If, in order to have a morally defensible health care delivery system, we must bring the masses up to the level of the fortunate few, we simply do not have the resources to do it. A middle course meets the moral demands while taking cognizance of the resource limitations.

WHOSE RESPONSIBILITY IS IT TO AFFECT CHANGE?

Stevens argues convincingly that nurses have an obligation to be involved in the national effort to reform our health care delivery system and to lobby for those currently outside the system or disadvantaged or wronged by it. This obligation extends beyond the responsibilities typically ascribed to a nurse. Traditionally, the scope of nurses' responsibilities has been limited to such things as loyalty to the physician with whom the nurse is working or advocacy for particular patients or clients. The nurse's responsibility has not always been seen as extending to those denied health care or to those who may need health care at some point in the future. A division of labor has been accepted whereby the nurse's role is circumscribed. The nurse qua nurse has fully exercised her or his responsibility when physicians' orders are properly executed and patients are adequately served.

Stevens rejects this view, holding nurses collectively responsible for working with others to shape a fairer and more humane health care delivery policy. The nurse's responsibilities are not exhausted by a review of her or his duties to particular patients and to associates in the workplace. These responsibilities extend as well to health-related matters of the society at large.

Stevens does not make explicit the basis for this wider responsibility. As I have argued elsewhere, the basis is to be found in the professional status of the nurse.[1] The nurse as professional joins with others to form a guild. In exchange for licensure and exclusive rights to practice nursing, nurses collectively have the responsibility to speak out on behalf of those in need of care and to promote among the public the benefits that derive from nursing research and knowledge.

As we move into the 21st century, the health care crisis looms large. If nurses as the largest single group of health care professionals recognize their collective responsibilities and turn their attention to this crisis, we stand a good chance of seeing some genuine advancements. We have Stevens to thank for the specific suggestions about how nurses can go about exercising their collective responsibility.

NOTE

[1] For a development of these arguments in favor of nurses' collective responsibility, see "The Nurse as a Member of a Profession," in James L. Muyskens, *Moral Problems in Nursing* [Totowa, NJ: Rowman and Littlefield], 1982.

Offprints. Requests for offprints should be sent to James Muyskens, Ph.D., 200 Strong Hall, University of Kansas, Lawrence, KS 66045-2100.

10

Equitable Access to Health Care: Continuing the Dialogue

Patricia E. Stevens, R.N., Ph.D.

School of Nursing
University of California, San Francisco

I acknowledge the editors of *Scholarly Inquiry for Nursing Practice: An International Journal*, especially Barbara Kos-Munson, for their commitment to improving health care access and thank the many respondents who reflected upon this important topic and shared their ideas with the nursing community. I join with them in the struggle to secure health care for all persons in the United States. In working toward a just health care system we are likely to disagree over values and strategy. I view such debate as a wellspring of empowerment, challenge, and insight. It is in this spirit that I continue the dialogue.

In considering access to care, it is imperative for us, as members of the nursing discipline, to situate our theory-building and policy-making in the everyday struggles of our clients, grounding our knowledge about health and health care in their worlds (Stevens & Hall, 1992). Under the structural conditions of the current U.S. system of health care delivery, clients' financial solvency is equated with deservedness. The profit motives of vast insurance, hospital, and medical industries encroach ever further upon the public's health as more and more exclusionary walls are put up to keep people from getting service. Clients are shut out, delegitimized, and exhausted in their battle to obtain health care. In addition to economic disenfranchisement, consumers face interactional obstacles. The trauma of gender, sexual orientation, ethnic, racial, and economic oppressions is not incidental, but chronic, insidious, and operative at the level of face-to-face health care interactions. As providers of health care, we are in more powerful positions than recipients. We have the responsibility for creating openness and receptivity in health care structures and health care interactions, rather than expecting clients to overcome myriad barriers to get taken care of properly.

I reaffirm even more urgently the challenge to nurses that we be the architects of a radically new structure of health care delivery in this country, one that makes comprehensive, nondiscriminatory health care universally available to everyone who lives in the United States. Since the article that opens this issue was written, the estimate of the numbers of uninsured people in the U.S. has risen from the commonly cited 35 million. The Bureau of the U.S. Census (1992) reports that as many as 61 million Americans are without health insurance for at least portions of the year. This figure suggests that one in four people lacks continuous health insurance coverage (Bovee, 1992). Sharp inequities along ethnic, racial, income, and age lines exist. Latinos, African Americans, low-income persons, inner-city dwellers, and the young are nearly twice as likely to lack health insurance.

IMPETUS FOR COMPREHENSIVE RESTRUCTURING

In his response to the article, Levine cautions against "feeling deeply about the inequities of our current non-system of health care delivery" because there is insufficient popular agreement, support, and organization to steer a course of action for change. Aroskar says that it is nearly impossible to change our current system until our society reaches consensus about what constitutes justice. Davis also suggests that we are stymied before we begin because the public will not pay. This favoring of inertia has been critiqued by Audre Lorde, an African American lesbian poet and essayist: "None of these struggles is ever easy. . . . It is so easy not to battle at all, to just accept, and to call that acceptance inevitable" (Lorde, 1988, p. 117).

As Levine indicates, there are formidable forces at work against a comprehensive restructuring of U.S. health care. The lobbying capabilities of the health insurance and medical industries are quite astounding. Over the past decade, the Political Action Committees of the Health Insurance Association of America, the American Medical Association, and other major insurance and medical organizations gave more than 19 million dollars in campaign contributions to lawmakers (Lee, 1992). These giants of political influence have persevered in their support of the status quo despite public opinion polls that consistently demonstrate deep-seated discontent with the U.S. health care system (Conine, 1990; Lipman, 1991; Morin, 1991; Scully, 1989; Steinbrook, 1990; Tuller, 1990). Insurance companies and physicians stand to lose significant entrepreneurial power in the emergence of a national health plan, especially one that is based on a single-payer model, so they have been steadfast in their objections.

The November 1991 upset victory of Pennsylvania Democrat Harris Wofford, however, appears to have changed the political tide. Wofford's promises of health care for all won him the U.S. Senate election (Chen, 1991; Russell, 1991). In the wake of this turn of events, the insurance and medical industries have had to acknowledge the public outcry for greater access and redirect their efforts to influence how that will be accomplished. Their preference is for incremental reforms that build on the current system and gradually extend coverage to more of the uninsured (Cohn, 1992).

THE REALITY OF INEQUITIES

Bonuck and Arno raise doubts that equity in health care distribution is a principle that Americans will endorse. Davis uses the word "utopian" to describe the premise that everyone has a right to health care. Muyskens asserts that standards of equitable access are too "high," that they "get in the way of a realistic approach" to the problems of health care. The institutional structures of health care in the United States reinforce physicians' powerful position over clients, maximize services for those who can afford them, and forsake significant segments of the population to endure avoidable pain, suffering, and death because of an inability to pay for health care (Baer, 1989; Caplan, 1989; Conners, 1980; Davis & Rowland, 1986; Mayster, Waitzkin, Hubbell, & Rucker, 1990). Is it overly idealistic to want to address these serious problems? Limited access to affordable, high-quality, appropriate, and nondiscriminatory health care results in diagnosis and treatment in later stages of illness and poorer prognosis for people of color, women, and the poor (Krieger, 1990; Saunders, 1989; Woolhandler & Himmelstein, 1989), which in the long run exacts a horrible individual and social cost. Is contending with such inequities anything other than facing reality? If we decide not to strive for equitable access in our systems of practice and distribution of services, the stakes are high for all, not only for the untold numbers of people who stand to lose their health, safety, and their very survival.

Rather than equity in health care access, Muyskens suggests a "decent minimum" of health services for all. Who decides what is a "decent minimum" of health care? Women? Children? People of color? Offering only the minimum to those who are "less fortunate" financially and politically would seem to preserve class, race, and gender stratification in this country. What is health promotion in a system that is built upon achieving the minimum?

NURSING'S AGENDA

With authors Joel, Betts, Moccia, and Aroskar, I applaud the American Nurses Association's document *Nursing's Agenda for Health Care Reform* (1991) for its strong stand in publicly asserting nursing's commitment to universal access to health care services, community-based primary care, illness prevention, and health promotion. Published after the article that opens this issue was written and submitted, *Nursing's Agenda* certainly demonstrates what I have called "nursing action to stem the spiraling decline in access to health care." The text of *Nursing's Agenda* recognizes that vulnerable groups within our society are denied access: ". . . millions of Americans must overcome enormous obstacles to get even the most elementary services" (p. 5). Countering Bonuck and Arno's argument that nurses do not experience the tension between meeting individual clients' health care needs and grappling with organizational resources that are insufficient for the task, the document points out that nurses witness the failings of the current health care system in the course of their everyday practice and ". . . see the alarming effects of a system that has lost touch with the communities it is supposed to serve" (p. 5). As Joel, Betts, Moccia, and Aroskar affirm, this document represents a fundamental belief of nurses that everyone should have access to high-quality nondiscriminatory health care. It also insists that major changes in the health care system be made now.

As a document that will be used to disseminate a specific policy for health care reform, *Nursing's Agenda* bears some examination. The plan set forth in the agenda calls for a combination of: (1) a government-run public health care system for people who are poor, uninsured, or ill (i.e., suffer from "preexisting conditions" that make them ineligible for private health care coverage), and (2) an insurance industry-run private health care system for people who can afford health insurance or are employed in jobs that offer benefits. The public system would make available a "federally defined standard package of essential health care services" (p. 2) to citizens and legal residents of the United States. The private system would offer the standard package plus "enriched" benefits and services.

I differ with Moccia's description of *Nursing's Agenda* as a "radical departure from the status quo." The plan seems to preserve the two-tiered health care system we presently have, differentiating the level of services once again by consumers' ability to pay rather than by health care needs. Comprehensive health care would be available only to those who are privileged members of the private system. Granted, the agenda stipulates expanded access to "essential services;" however, the components of this "standard package of essential health care services" remain unspecified.

A health care plan consistent with the aims of nursing would reflect consideration of the ethics involved in institutionalized rationing of services to low-income and ill consumers who cannot purchase "enriched" health care services. *Nursing's Agenda* ought to begin, not with the assumption that there are no alternatives to rationing, but with an examination of all options, many of which are currently in place in the health care systems of other countries. Doesn't the importance and constancy of need for health care suggest a more permanent nurse-managed, stably funded network of services that cannot be fiscally exploited to fund other political needs?

Nursing's Agenda seems to further reinforce the profit-making corporate organization of health care by posing tasks to consumers that have proved backbreaking if not impossible under the current system: (1) "public funding for extended care if consumer resources are exhausted" (p. 4), (2) "emphasis on consumers' responsibility to financially plan for their long-term care needs" (p. 4) through home equity conversion plans and the like, (3) elimination of payment at the time of service and elimination of balance billing (p. 4), but no protection from accumulation of overwhelming health care debt, and (4) consumer responsibility for premiums, deductibles, and copayments in both the public system and the private system to serve as "financial incentives to be economical in their use of services" (p. 13). The agenda assures that these provisions "will never serve as barriers to care" (p. 13), a promise that is empty and illogical at best. Having one's savings exhausted, losing one's home to pay for long-term care, becoming dependent on friends, family, and perhaps the state because of massive health care debts are all enormous threats for the majority of people in the United States.

Placing the costs of premiums, deductibles, and copayments upon individuals is always disproportionately burdensome for those with low incomes and often forestalls seeking of needed care.

Nursing's Agenda strives to "preserve the best elements of the existing system" (p. 5). By perpetuating the conglomeration of 1500 private insurance companies (Russo, 1991), a for-profit hospital industry, and a relatively unregulated medical profession, many of whose members garner extraordinary personal incomes with their fees-for-service, one might reasonably argue that the *Agenda* preserves the worst elements of the existing system. I am critical of the *Agenda* because it is directed toward obtaining a modicum of expanded access to health care without calling into question major elements of the existing system. In effect, by appeasing the powerbrokers and avoiding overt political conflict, organized nursing is taking a stance that may ultimately forsake diverse groups of consumers in desperate need of a strong advocate.

CONCLUSION

Our nursing organizations are a powerful base from which we as a profession can influence national policy. To make our organizational voice effective and pertinent to the daily struggles of health care consumers and practicing nurses, we must take action and speak out about what we envision for the public's health. Open debate about whose interests we favor in seeking changes in the U.S. health care system will clarify our positions. Specific attention to access in our research and intervention will give us empirical and clinical evidence. By personally advising our constituent nursing organizations about the direction we want the profession to take in the national debate, nurses can ensure that organizational stances reflect our experiences and sentiments.

As nurses, our numbers and centuries of direct caregiving experience have earned us the right to speak about this health care crisis. We are not of a single voice. As a discipline, nursing has evolved to a point where diversity of views is not only tolerated, but considered a strength. Nursing organizations need to seize this opportunity to negotiate a coalition within nursing and with consumers that will effect major, tangible changes in health care in the U.S.

REFERENCES

American Nurses Association. (1991). *Nursing's agenda for health care reform*. Kansas City, MO: American Nurses Publishing.

Baer, H. A. (1989). The American dominative medical system as a reflection of social relations in the larger society. *Social Science and Medicine, 28*(11), 1103–1112.

Bovee, T. (1992, June 25). 25% of Americans lack health insurance. *San Francisco Examiner*, p. 13.

Caplan, R. L. (1989). The commodification of American health care. *Social Science and Medicine, 28*(11), 1139–1148.

Chen, E. (1991, November 8). Survey finds health care top vote issue. *Los Angeles Times*, p. 26.

Cohn, V. (1992, January 21). Moving on health care reform: The challenge to the President and Congress. *The Washington Post*, p. 210.

Conine, E. (1990, March 26). Canada's sensible approach: While U.S. politicians recoil at the mention of national insurance, our neighbors to the north are becoming the envy of many Americans. *Los Angeles Times*, p. B7.

Connors, D. D. (1980). Sickness unto death: Medicine as mythic, necrophilic and iatrogenic. *Advances in Nursing Science, 2*(3), 39–51.

Davis, K., & Rowland, D. (1986). Uninsured and underserved: Inequities in health care in the United States. In P. Conrad & R. Kern (Eds.), *The sociology of health and illness: Critical perspectives* (pp. 250–266). New York: St. Martin's Press.

Krieger, N. (1990). Racial and gender discrimination: Risk factors for high blood pressure? *Social Science and Medicine, 30*(12), 1273–1281.

Lee, G. (1992, March 16). Health insurance lobby mounts effort against adoption of Canadian system. *The Washington Post*, p. 15.

Lipman, L. (1991, April 8). Health care hits the critical list. *The Atlanta Journal and Constitution*, p. 1.

Lorde, A. (1988). *A burst of light*. Ithaca, NY: Firebrand Books.

Mayster, V., Waitzkin, H., Hubbell, F. A, & Rucker, L. (1990). Local advocacy for the medically indigent: Strategies and accomplishments in one county. *Journal of the American Medical Association, 263*(2), 262–268.

Morin, R. (1991, December 31). Americans grade their health care. *The Washington Post*, p. Z6.

Russell, S. (1991, November 12). Health care reformers clash at Berkeley forum: National insurance movement highlighted. *San Francisco Chronicle*, p. 7.

Russo, M. (1991, December 24). Universal health care plan overdue. *Chicago Tribune*, p. 10.

Saunders, L. D. (1989). Differences in the timeliness of diagnosis of breast and cervical cancer, San Francisco 1974–85. *American Journal of Public Health, 79*(1), 69–73.

Scully, M. (1989, September 8). Americans favor tax for health insurance—up to a point. *The Washington Times*, p. C10.

Steinbrook, R. (1990, February 4). Majority favors reform of U.S. health care system. *Los Angeles Times*, p. 1.

Stevens, P. E., & Hall, J. M. (1992). Applying critical theories to nursing in communities. *Public Health Nursing, 9*(1), 2–9.

Tuller, D. (1990, May 3). Poll shows wide support on health care for poor. *San Francisco Chronicle*, p. 9.

U.S. Bureau of the Census. (1992). Health insurance coverage: 1987 to 1990. *Current Population Report* (Series P-70, No. 29). Washington, DC: U.S. Government Printing Office.

Woolhandler, S., & Himmelstein, D. U. (1989). Ideology in medical science: Class in the clinic. *Social Science and Medicine, 28*(11), 1205–1209.

Acknowledgment. The author wishes to acknowledge Joanne M. Hall, R.N., Ph.D., Postdoctoral Fellow, School of Nursing U.C.S.F., for her critical and conceptual support in preparing this response.

Offprints. Requests for offprints should be sent to Patricia E. Stevens, R.N., Ph.D., 1612 Noriega Street, San Francisco, CA 94122.

11

A Summary of Nursing's Agenda for Health Care Reform

America's nurses have long supported the restructuring of our Nation's health care system with the goal of assuring access, quality, and affordable cost. The components of a basic "core of services" to be made available to all include:

- Consumer access to care through primary health services delivered in community-based settings.
- Consumer responsibility for the personal health, self care, and informed decision-making in selecting health care services.
- Utilization of the most cost-effective providers and therapeutic options in appropriate settings.

A federally defined standard package of essential health services for all citizens and residents is called for, provided and financed through an integration of public and private plans and sources and including:

- A public plan based on federal guidelines and eligibility requirements providing coverage for the poor.
- The opportunity for small businesses and individuals, particularly those at risk because of preexisting conditions, and those potentially medically indigent, to buy into the plan.
- A private plan offering, at a minimum, the nationally standardized package of essential services.

This package can be enhanced as a benefit of employment or individually purchased. A phase-in of essential services shall include:

- Coverage of pregnant women and children.
- Assistance to vulnerable populations who have had limited access to health care.

Planned change is required which attends to health care needs correlated to changing National demographics including:

- Incentives for both consumers and providers to utilized managed care approaches.

• Incentives for cost-effectiveness.
• Controlled growth of the system through prudent planning and resource allocation.
• Policy development based on outcomes research.
• Assurance of qualified providers.

A case management based system accompanied by an active advocacy program is required for those with continuing health needs and includes:

• Assured public and private funding for services, both short and long-term.
• Emphasis on consumer participation in financial planning.
• Insurance reform.
• Establishment of review policies and procedures in both public and private sectors.

SP *Springer Publishing Company*

NURSING CARE OF THE PATIENT WHO SMOKES

Patricia G. Rienzo, RN, BSN

The purpose of the book is to make nurses more aware of the health implications of tobacco smoking and to help them develop interventions to assist smokers to cease smoking, to discourage initiation of smoking among young people, and to improve the quality of health care provided to smokers.

Contents: Smoking, a Problem for Nurses • Smoking and Disease • Understanding Smoking Behavior • Helping Smokers Quit • Pharmacological Adjuncts to Smoking Cessation • Nursing Care of the Ill Smoker • Smoking and Nutrition • Drug Interactions and Tobacco Smoking • The Nurse Who Smokes • Prevention of Tobacco Smoking • Social, Political, Legal, Economic and Ethical Aspects of Tobacco Use

1992 216pp 0-8261-7620-8 hard $29.95 (outside US $33.80)

536 Broadway • New York, NY 10012 • (212) 431- 4370 • Fax: (212) 941-7842